Examination of the Neurological System

M.Ismail MD

First Published, 2016

ISBN: 1539570185
ISBN-13: 978-1539570189

DEDICATION

To every student of medicine that will learn to appreciates this simple fact – no matter how helpful this book may be, the ultimate teacher will always be your patient.

Contents

Introduction:

This book is simple. This is not one of those thick medical textbooks filled with long paragraphs that put you to sleep faster than a general anaesthetic. No. Instead, this book respects the fact that as a med student or doctor your time is precious. Every minute counts.

Saying that let me take 33 seconds to explain what this book is about:
It will comprehensively guide you through the entire neurological examination, including the mental state, motor, sensory, cranial nerve and cerebellar systems. Almost every technique is accompanied by a step-wise approach as well as clear images depicting exactly how to do it.

Since examinations require practice to perfect, this handbook can be easily stored in your backpack, handbag or white coat. It will then always be at hand to learn, practise and improve on your technique of examining the neurological system.

Also, right at the end there is a summary of everything neatly squashed on to a few pages for you to revise from.

So go grab that blue and red energy drink and let's get examining!

M.Ismail MD

Overview of the Neurological Examination

There are 5 different examinations:
   1.) The Mental State Exam
   2.) The Motor System
   3.) The Sensory System
   4.) The Cranial Nerves
   5.) The Cerebellar System

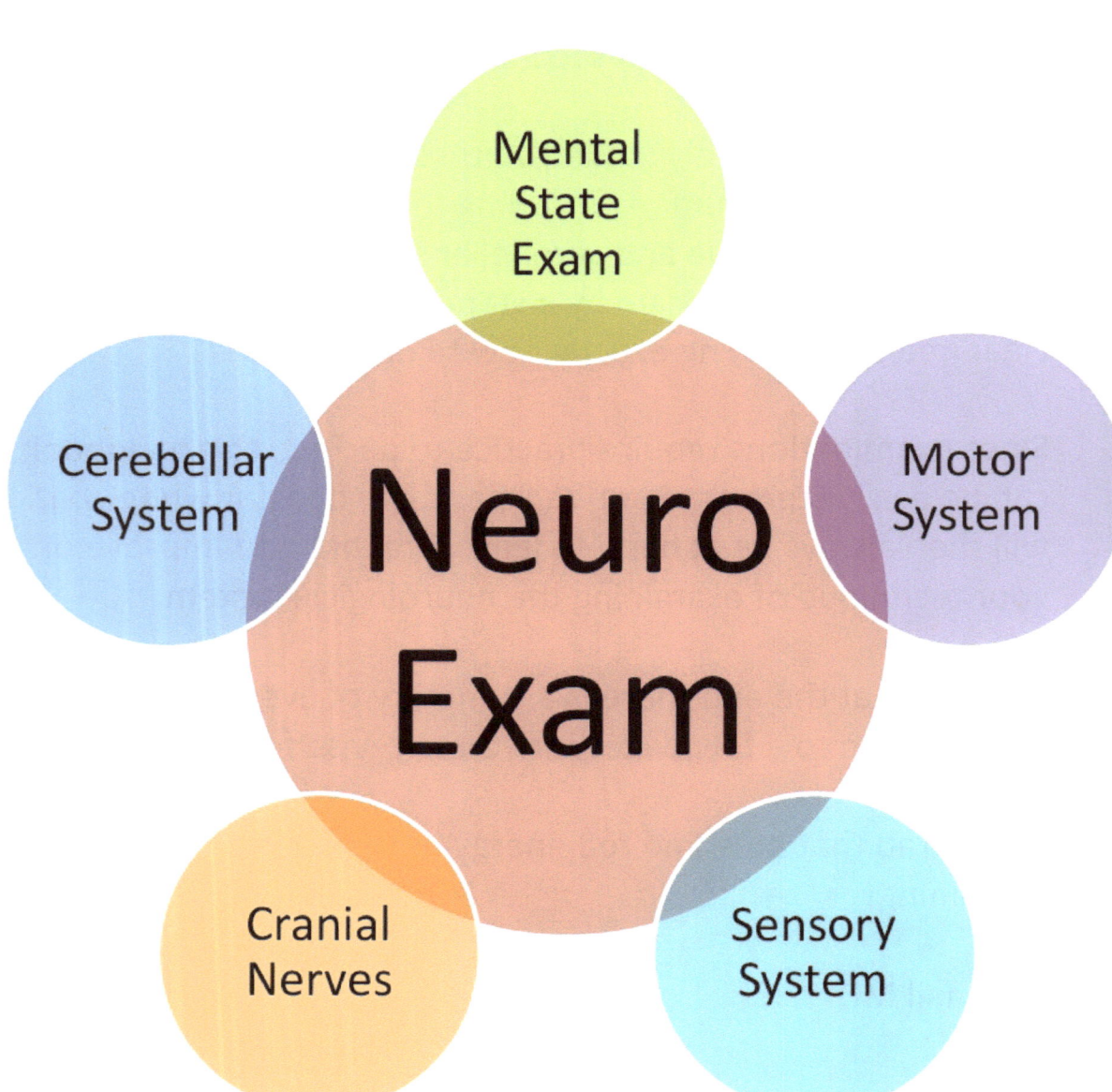

Chapter 1

The Mental State Examination (MSE)

- The first part of the MSE involves assessing the consciousness of the patient
- **Consciousness** is checked using the **Glasgow Coma Scale (GCS)**

The Glasgow Coma Scale (GCS):

Eye Opening	Spontaneous	4
	To speech	3
	To pain	2
	None	1
Verbal Response	Orientated 5	
	Confused/disoriented 4	
	Inappropriate words 3	
	Incomprehensible sounds 2	
	None 1	
Motor	Obeys commands 6	
	Localizes pain 5	
	Withdraws from pain 4	
	Abnormal flexion to pain 3	
	Extension to pain 2	
	None 1	

Note: The lowest score of the GCS is 3/15, unless the patient is intubated in which case, the patient is assessed as being 2T/15

Top Tip:
When assessing a patient start from the top of the patient's body (Eyes, scored out of 4), then move down (to the Mouth, scored out of 5), then down to the rest of the body (to the Motor System, scored out of 6)

MMSE (Mini Mental State Exam)

- The easiest way to test mental state is with the MMSE (mini mental state exam)
- This tool gives a rough guideline on the type of questions needed to perform a mental state exam
- It is scored as follows:

1.) Orientation	10
2.) Language: name and repetition	3
3.) Registration	3
4.) Attention/concentration/calculation	5
5.) Recall	3
6.) Language: reading comprehension	1
7.) Praxis	3
8.) Praxis and Language	1
9.) Praxis and visuo-spatial ability	1
Total:	30

- The total maximum score on the MMSE is 30 points
- A score of less than 24 points is suggestive of dementia or delirium

Note:
The MMSE does not need to be done on each and every neurological patient, but should be done if there is a concern that the patient may be suffering from delirium/dementia

MMSE

1.) Orientation

- What day of the week is it?   1

- What is the date today?
    o Day   1
    o Month   1
    o Year   1

- What is the season?   1

- In what country are we?   1

- In which province are we?   1

- What is the name of this city?   1

- In which building are we?   1

- On which floor are we?   1

                                             (10)

2.)Name and repetition:

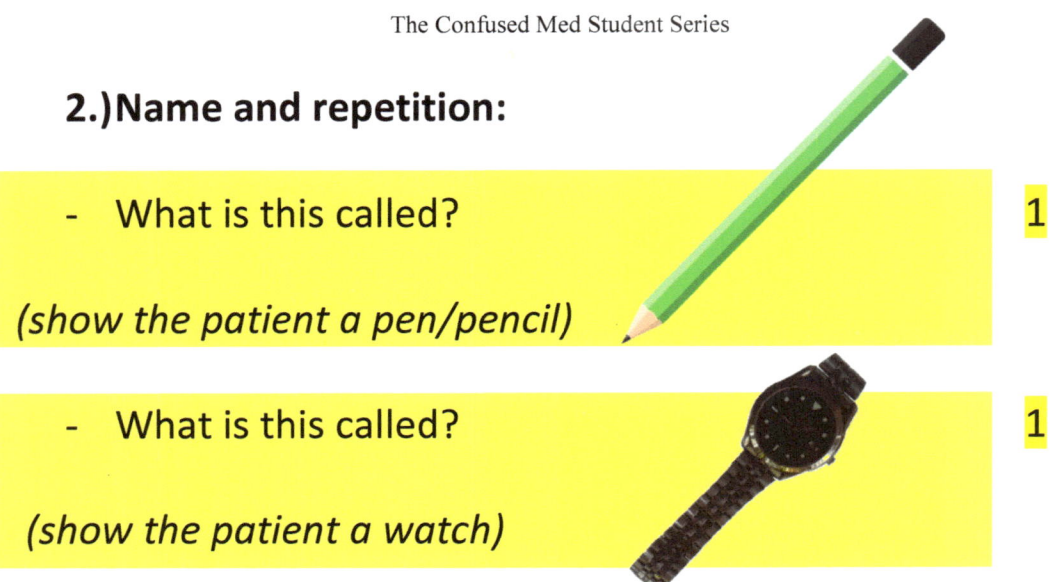

- What is this called?   1

(show the patient a pen/pencil)

- What is this called?   1

(show the patient a watch)

- I am going to say something, I would like you to repeat it after me:
    "No ifs, ands or buts"   1

                                                        (3)

3.)Registration:

"Now I am going to name 3 objects.
After I have finished saying all three, I want you to repeat them. Remember what they are, because I am going to ask you to name them again in a few minutes"

Say clearly:
- APPLE   1
- TABLE   1
- PEN   1

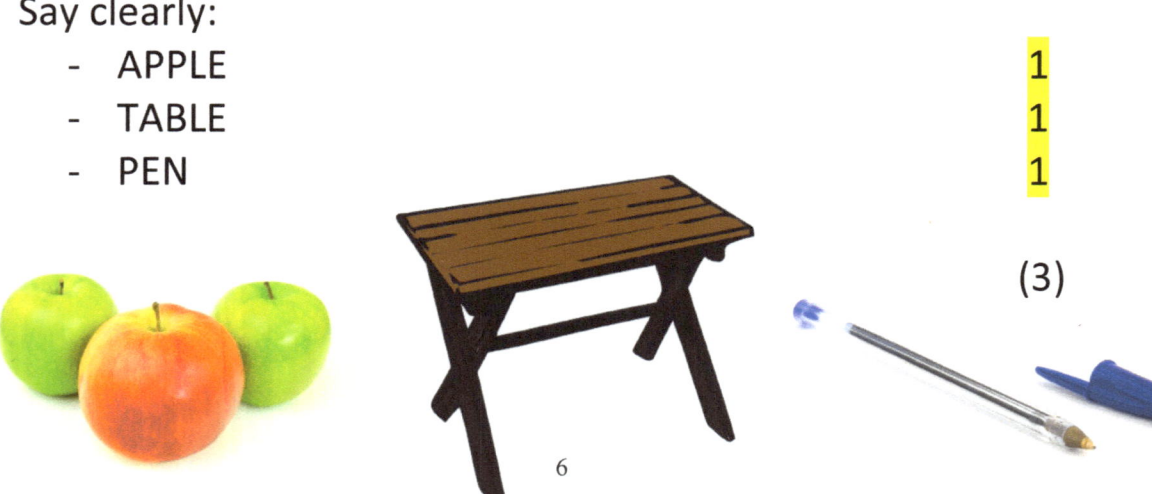

                                                        (3)

4.)Attention/calculation

"Now I would like you to take away or subtract 7 from 100. Then take away another 7 and continue subtracting 7 until I ask you to stop."

100	93	86	79	72	65
1	1	1	1	1	1

OR

"Spell the word WORLD backwards"

D	L	R	O	W
1	1	1	1	1

5.)Recall:

"What were the three objects I asked you to repeat a little while ago?"

- APPLE   1
- TABLE   1
- PEN   1

6.)Reading comprehension:

"Read this page and do what it says."   1

Close Your Eyes

7.) Praxis:

"I am going to give you a piece of paper. When I do, take it with your right hand, fold it in half with both hands and put it down on your lap."

- Right hand   1
- Folds paper   1
- Puts on lap   1

8.) Praxis and Language:

"Please write a complete sentence of your choice on this piece of paper"   1

9.) Praxis and visuo-spatial ability

"Copy this design"   1

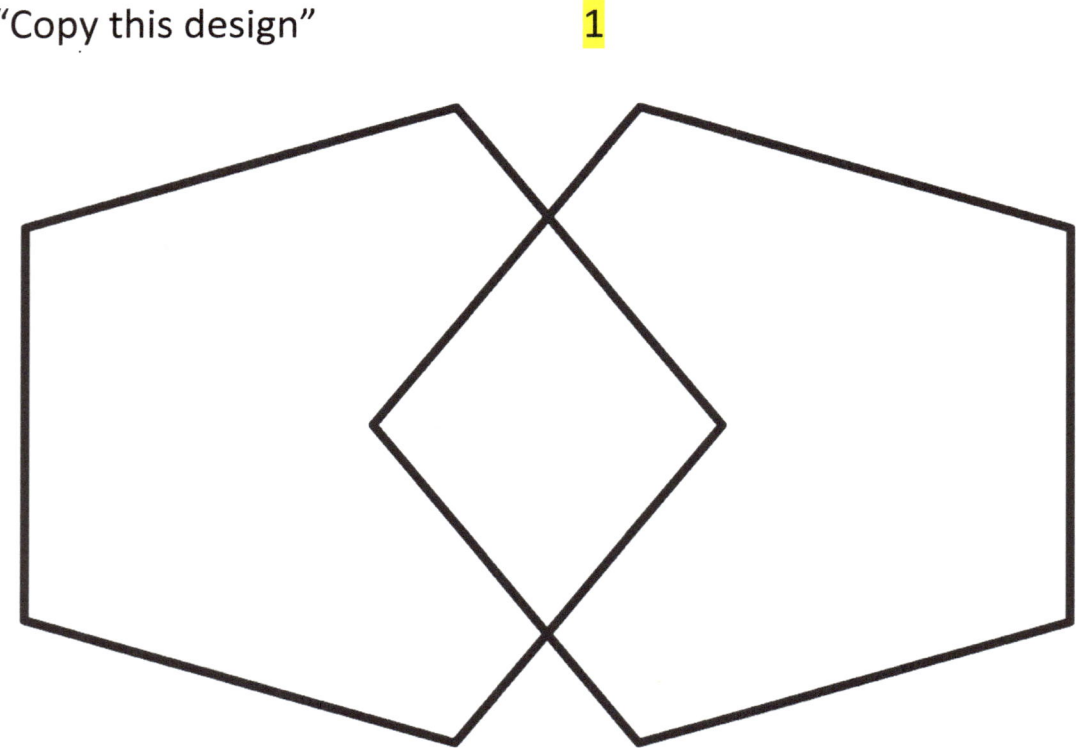

Chapter 2

The Motor System

- This system is divided as follows:
  - o Inspection
  - o Tone
  - o Power
  - o Reflexes

Inspection

- **Check for wasting**
    - In other words, check for muscle bulk
    - There are 2 scenarios where you would have wasting (decreased muscle bulk):
        - Lack of use/disuse of the muscle
            - This occurs over months
            - Similar to when you don't go to gym for a few months
        - Neurogenic wasting
            - When the nerve supplying the muscle is severed
            - This type of wasting occurs quickly
            - Occurs over days to weeks

- **Check for any abnormal twitches**
    - These are Known as **fasciculations**
    - Occurs in LMN (lower motor neuron) disease
    - It is when the muscle spontaneously discharges and contracts

- **Check for deformity**
    - E.g. Foot Drop:
        - Dropping of the forefoot due to weakness
        - There is an inability to dorsiflex the foot up
        - May be a sign of paralysis of the leg

    - E.g. clawing of the hand
        - Indicates weakness of the ulnar muscle

Tone
Definition:
- Mild resistance in healthy muscle

Method for assessing tone:
<mark>Upper Limbs:</mark>
- Arms:
  - <mark>**Supinate and pronate the arm**</mark>
  - Feel the resistance
  - Ask the patient to relax!
  - Check both arms
  - Note: Supination is affected more than pronation in the case of increased tone!

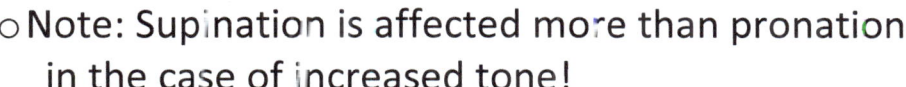

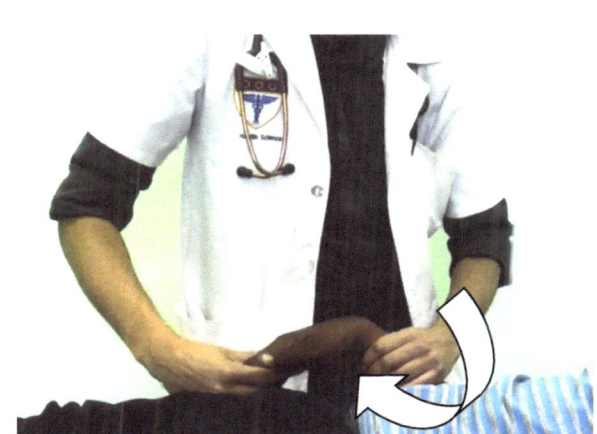

- Wrist:
  - <mark>**Circumduct the wrist to check for tone**</mark>
  - Do this on both wrists

- Arms:
  - <mark>**Flex and extend**</mark> the arm backwards and forwards

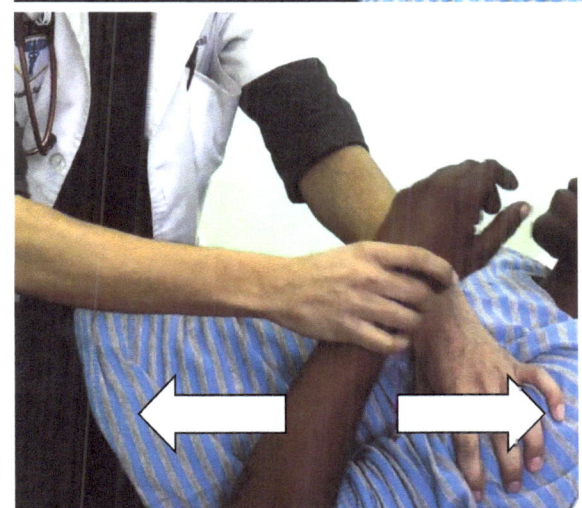

<mark>Lower Limbs:</mark>

- Legs:
  - Shake the leg forward and backwards a bit and look at the ankle joint – it normally should have a bit of a wobble
  - This is known as <mark>log-rolling the leg</mark>

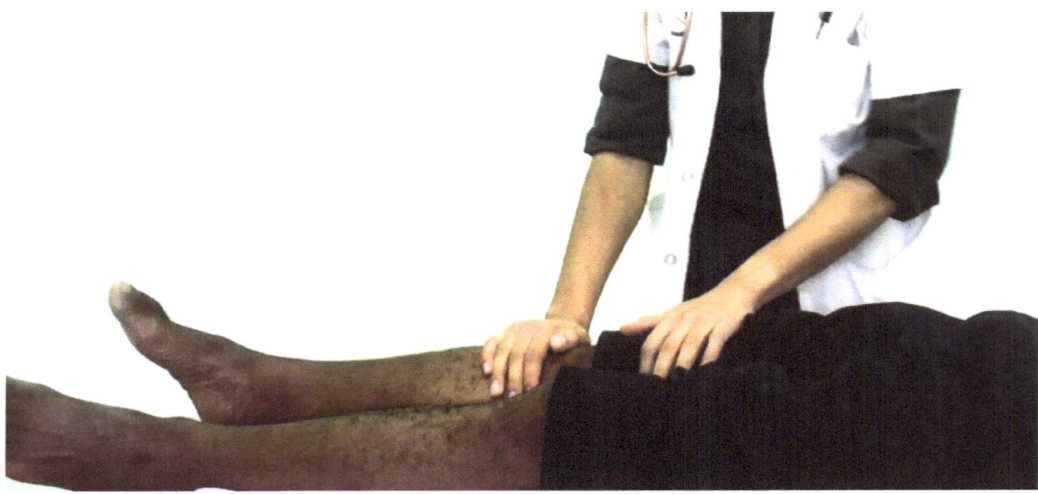

  - Another method to assess lower limb tone:
    - Lift the leg/thigh up quickly under the knee
    - If the ankle lifts off bed then there's ↑ tone
    - If the ankle slides on the bed then there's normal tone (this stretches the quadriceps)

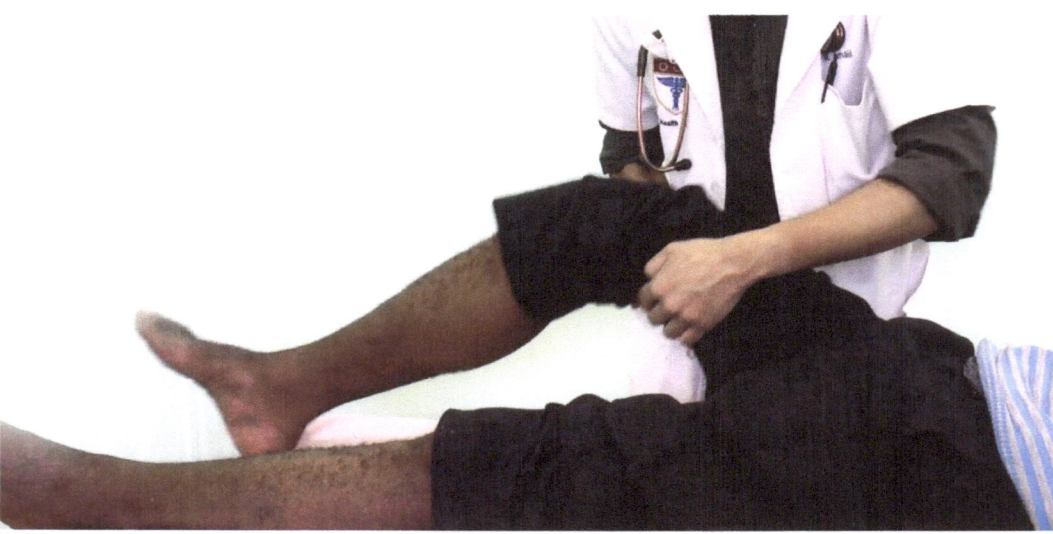

==Pathology of tone:==
- Either 1 of two possibilities:
  o Hypertonia (usually Upper Motor Neuron Lesion)
    OR   (UMN)
  o Hypotonia (usually Lower Motor Neuron Lesion)
                    (LMN)

1.) Hypertonia
- 2 types:
  o ==Rigidity (extra-pyramidal disease e.g. Parkinsons)==
    ▪ Mild stiffness over all the muscles
    ▪ Sometimes referred to as **cogwheel rigidity**
      • (because of its bump-bump-bump nature as resistance comes and fades all the time)
      • Can check by circumducting the wrist
  o ==Spasticity (corticospinal disease e.g. Motor Neuron Disease)==
    ▪ Can't change tone quickly!
    ▪ If you try and quickly move a muscle it locks against you
      • This is known as a **spastic catch**
    ▪ But if you gently open it, and it is a bit stiff
      • This is known as **clasp-knife**

==Clonus:==
- This sign may accompany spasticity
- It is also an UMN sign
- One can check for ankle clonus and knee clonus

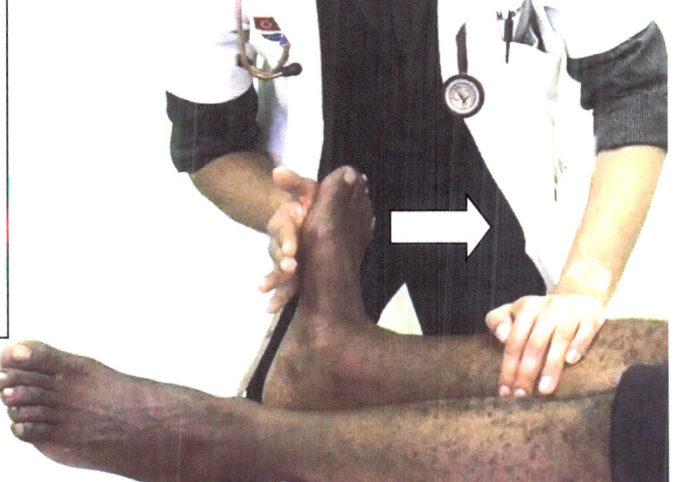

Power

<mark>Note: always position the muscle in the expected position and then try and resist it</mark>
- i.e. if you want to test bicep flexion, start with the biceps flexed already; if you want to test triceps extension then extend the arms first before applying resistance

Power is graded according to the following criteria:

0/5	No muscular contractions
1/5	Flicker of muscular contraction
2/5	Movement but not against gravity
3/5	Movement against gravity
4/5	Some resistance against movement
5/5	Full power/resistance against movement

Myotomes
- Each group of muscles is supplied by nerves that send information from the motor cortex in the brain
- These nerves exit the spinal cord at different spinal cord levels (e.g. C5, C6 etc)
- A myotome is defined as a group of muscles supplied by single spinal nerve root (i.e. a group of muscles supplied by nerves exiting at specific spinal cord levels)
- The motor examination is guided by the understanding of myotomes as can be seen below
- Each part of the examination assesses these different spinal cord levels

Method:

Upper Limb:
==C5:==
- ==**Deltoids**==
  - Ask patient to put both arms up and ask to resist when you push down on deltoids
  - Press down on the shoulders/deltoids and assess the power
  - Normal: you can't budge the arms down

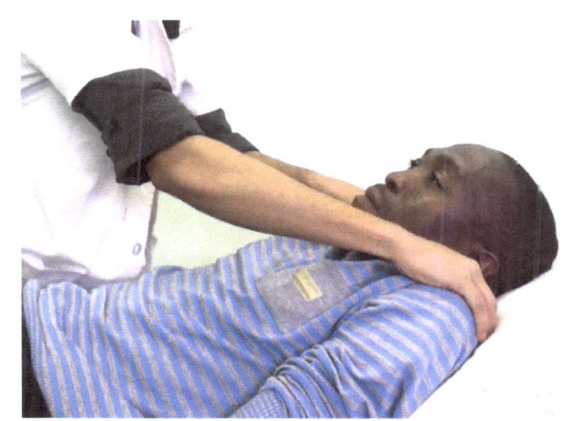

==C6:==
- ==**Biceps:**==
  - Compare right with left
  - Normal: you can't budge the arms
  - Start with the arm flexed

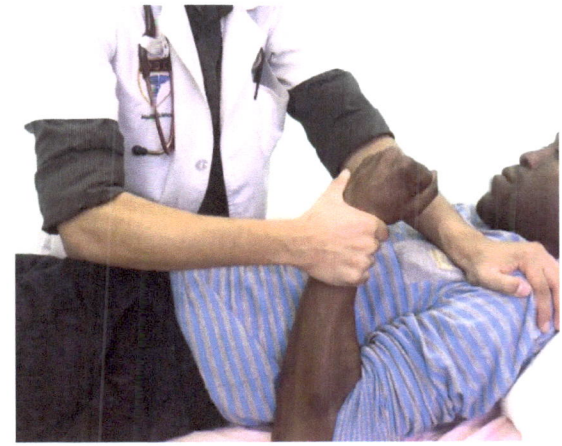

==C7:==
- ==**Triceps:**==
  - Compare right with left
  - Normal: you can't budge the arms
  - Start with the arm extended

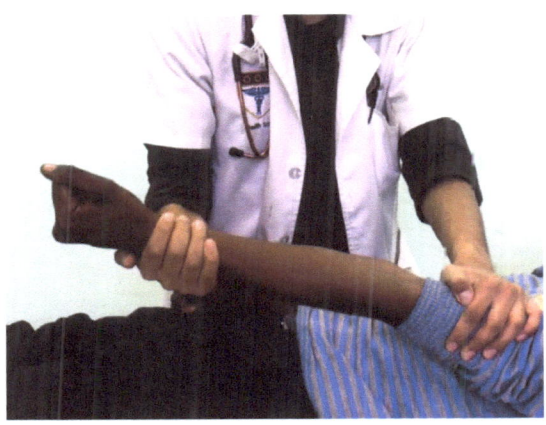

C8:

- **Grip:**
  - Give patient **2 of your fingers** to grip as tight as they can
  - Compare right with left (in other words give both your fingers at the same time)

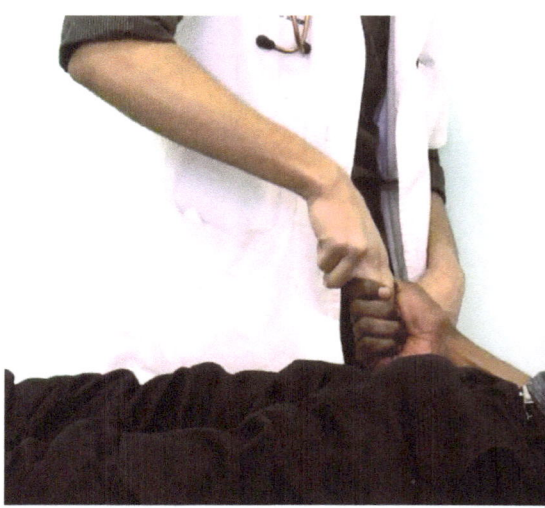

T1:

- **Fingers abducted:**
  - Ensure the patient's fingers are open with all five fingers separated and level with the ground
  - Then squeeze the index and little finger gently towards each other
  - Compare resistance between right and left

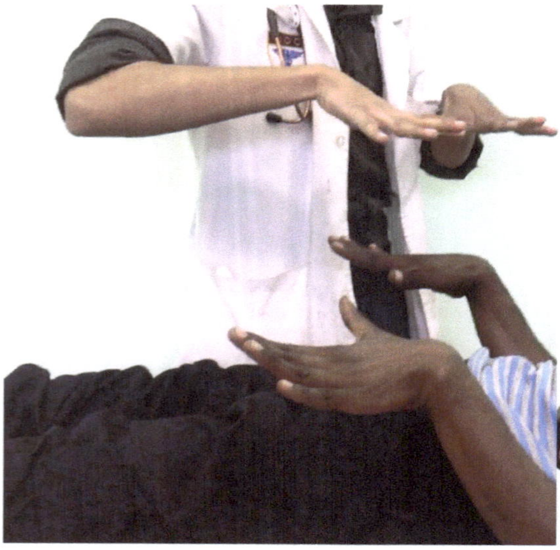

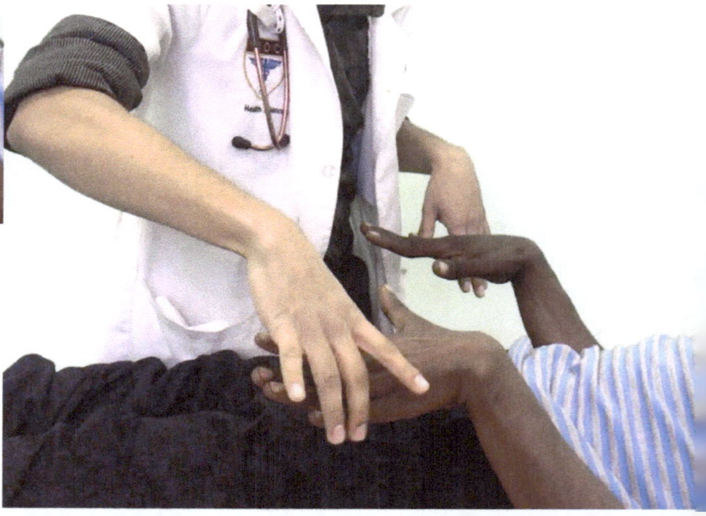

Lower Limbs:

<mark>L2:</mark>
- **Hip Flexion (Iliopsoas)**
  - o Ask the patient to bend their knee and bring their leg up
  - o This is hip flexion, therefore once it is in this position you can try and resist it in order to assess the power

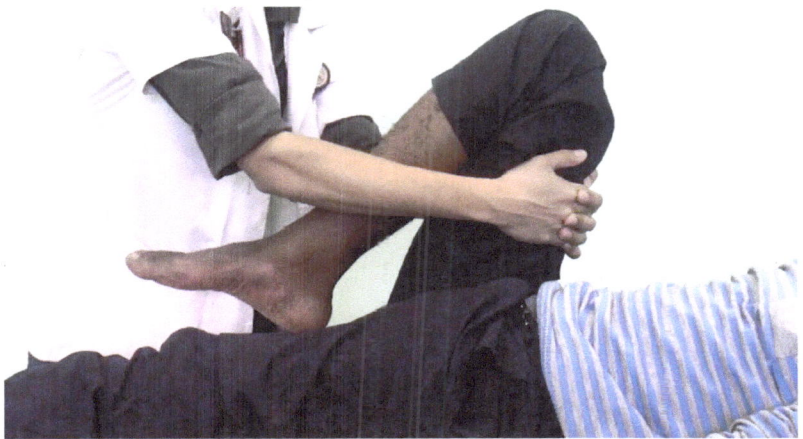

<mark>L3:</mark>
- **Knee Extension (Quadriceps)**
  - o Lift leg up and straighten it out
  - o Then ask patient to keep it stiff
  - o Try and budge it to assess power

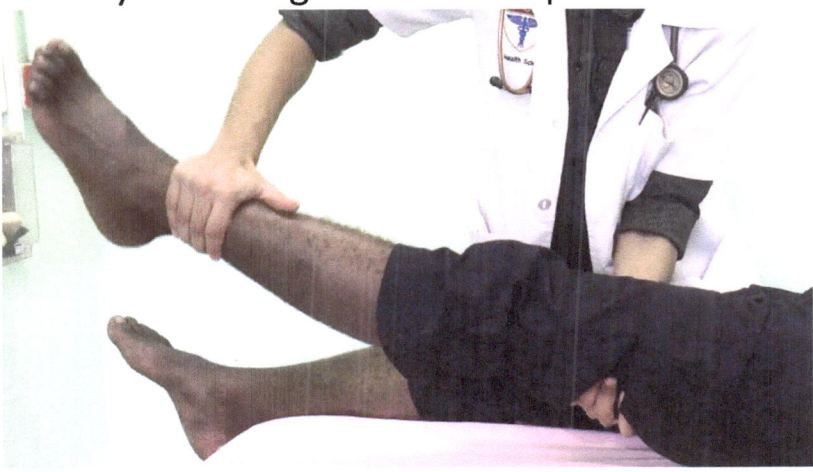

L4:

- **Ankle Dorsiflexion (Tibialis Anterior)**
  - Ask patient to point ankles up (dorsiflex foot)
  - Then try and budge it downwards
  - Ensure that you check both ankles!

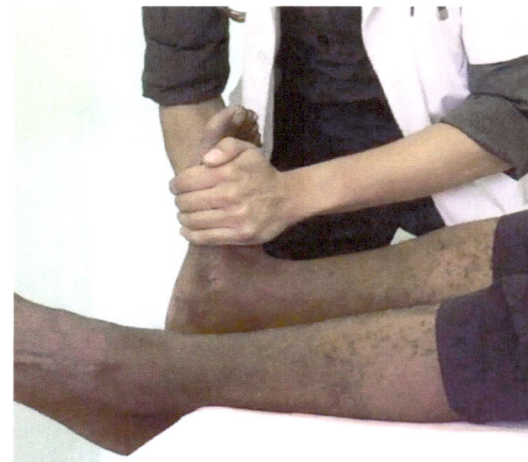

L5:

- **Big Toe Extension**
  - Ask patient to point big toe upwards
  - Can usually overcome this but with a bit of resistance though

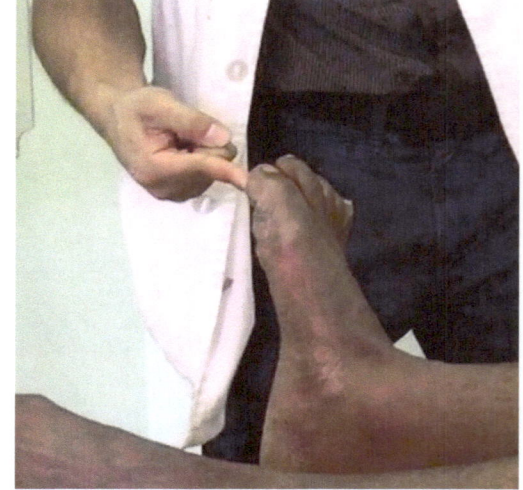

S1:

- **Plantar Flexion**
  - Ask patient to point foot downwards
  - Try and budge by pushing up against it
  - This is a very strong muscle therefore it shouldn't budge at all

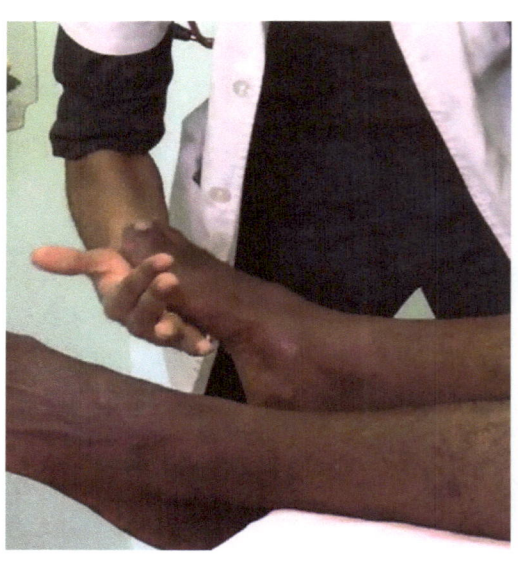

Trunk:

Inspect:
- ==Abdominal Muscles:==
    - **Ask patient to bring their head off the bed (therefore patient will tense his rectus abdominus muscles)**
    - Normal: umbilicus remains in position
    - If paralysed from the abdomen down: the muscles below the umbilicus will be weak and the muscles above the umbilicus would tense - this would result in the umbilicus rising up when the patient lifts his head off the bed!

- ==Paradoxical Breathing:==
    - **Occurs when the diaphragm is paralyzed**
    - Normal: the diaphragm moves downwards on inspiration (as it contracts)
    - If paralyzed: the diaphragm rises into the chest on inspiration

Tendon Reflexes

- What are we doing?
  - o We are **stretching** the tendon with the hammer and reflexly it will contract
  - o Therefore:
    - The position we put the limb in will affect the reflex!
    - The position we should put the limb in, is in a slightly stretched position.
    - The right side and the left side must be in a similar position

---

4 possibilities of reflexes:
1.) Normal
2.) Decreased, but present
3.) Absent
4.) Hyper-reflexic

Upper Limb:

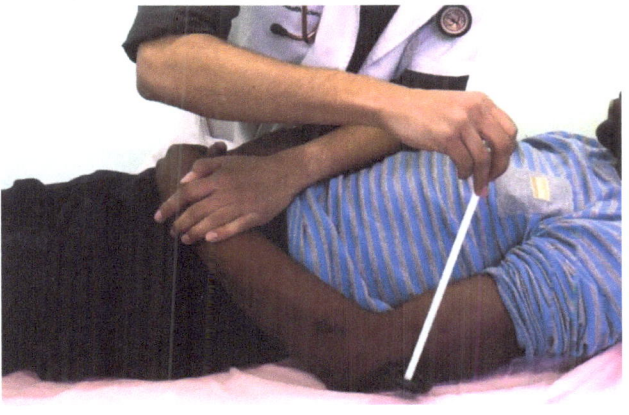

<mark>Biceps Reflex (C5, C6):</mark>

- Position the arms as follows:
    - Both arms slightly bent and resting on the abdomen
- Finding the tendon:
    - The biceps tendon is on the medial side of the anticubital fossa
    - Place your finger on the tendon
    - Gently tap with the patella hammer
- The reflex:
    - Watch the biceps muscle for contraction
    - Feel the tendon for the contraction as well

<mark>Triceps Reflex (C7):</mark>

- Position the arms as follows:
    - Let the arm lie on the trunk
    - If you want him relaxed, you must let him take the weight of his arm
- Finding the tendon:
    - Triceps is a broad tendon, so you won't miss it
    - Gently tap directly onto the tendon with the patella hammer just above the elbow
- The reflex:
    - Watch the triceps muscle for contraction

Supinator Reflex (brachioradialis muscle – C5, C6):

- Position the arms as follows:
    - o Both arms slightly bent and resting on the abdomen (same as in biceps position)

- Finding the tendon:
    - o Tap directly onto the muscle on the lateral side of the arm
    - o Gently tap with the patella hammer

- The reflex:
    - o Watch the brachioradialis muscle (forearm) for contraction
    - o Usually not a very prominent reflex therefore you don't usually see much

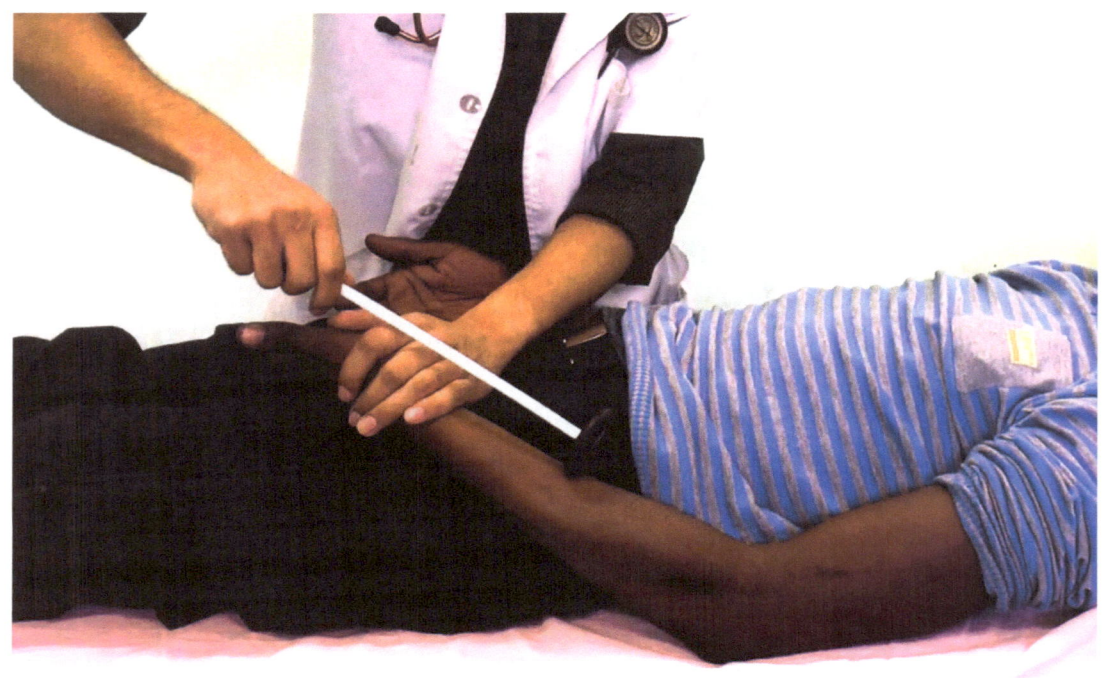

Lower Limb:

<mark>Knee Reflex (L4):</mark>

- Position the legs as follows:
    - o Support the leg and bend the knee slightly
    - o The leg can be supported by placing your arm under the leg and resting your hand on the opposite thigh
- Finding the tendon:
    - o The patella is in the tendon
    - o Therefore feel for the tendon below the patella (1cm wide)
    - o Gently tap with the patella hammer
    - o Always compare with the opposite side
- The reflex:
    - o Watch the quadriceps muscle for contraction
    - o This is one of the more obvious of the reflexes

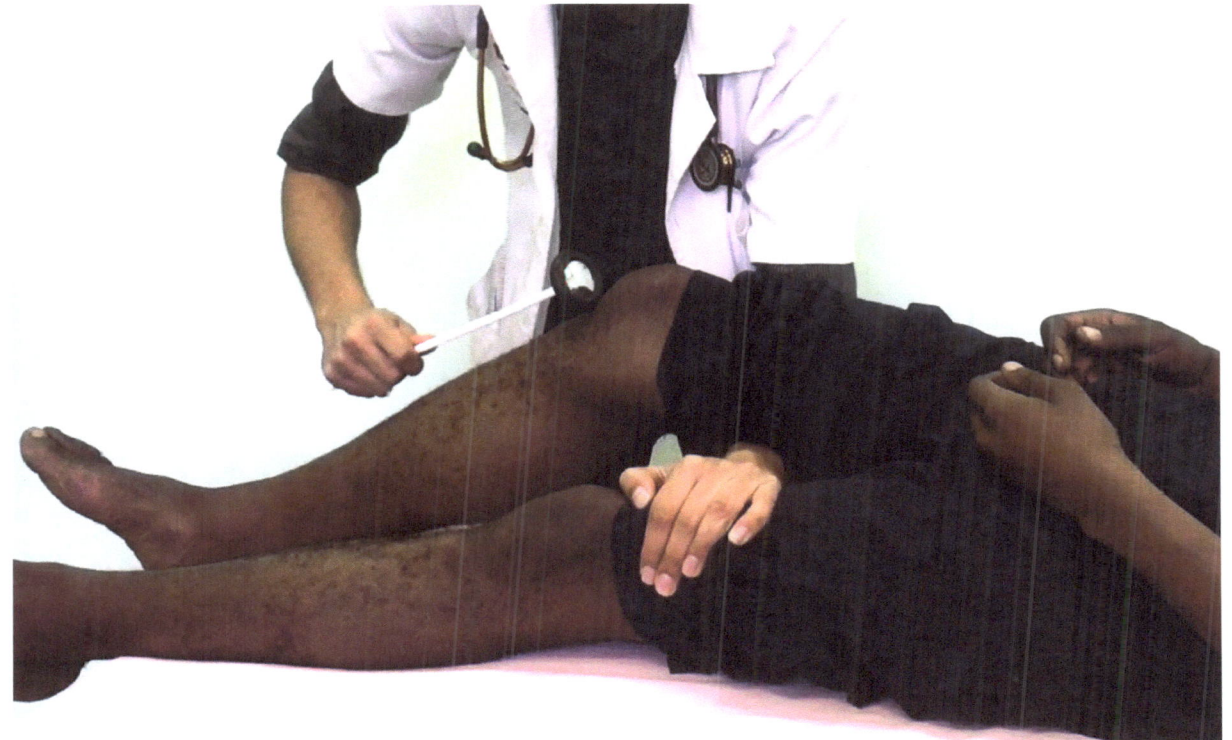

Ankle Reflex (S1):

- Position the legs as follows (technique is NB here!):
    - Bend the knee out laterally
    - **Place your fingers under the foot and pull the foot up so that you gently stretch the calf muscle (fully!)**
    - Place your thumb on the top of the foot (to stop patient from interfering)
- Finding the tendon:
    - The tendon will be stretched whilst in this position and is found just above the heel
    - Gently tap with the patella hammer
    - Always compare with the opposite side
- The reflex:
    - Watch for contraction in the calf muscle

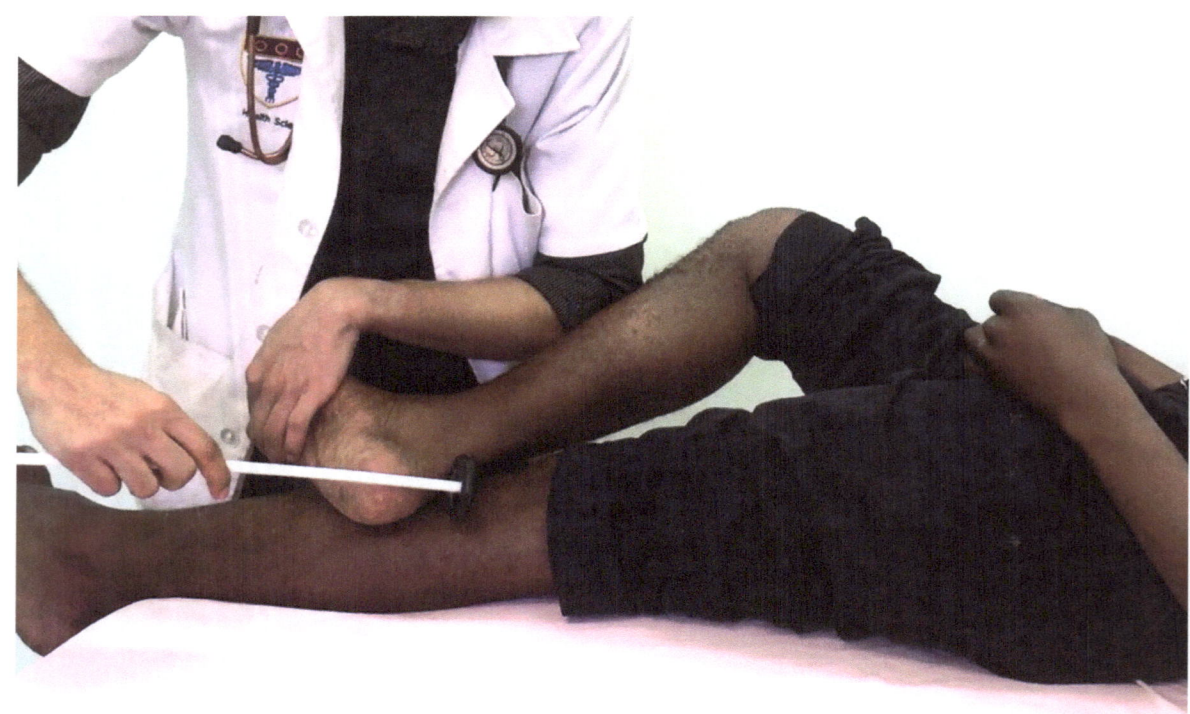

Plantar Reflex (S1, S2):

- Important in UMN Disease
- How to do the reflex:
    - Use a blunt object (e.g. your thumb) that is not painful nor ticklish
    - Start at base of foot, run it up the lateral side of the foot and then just below the toes

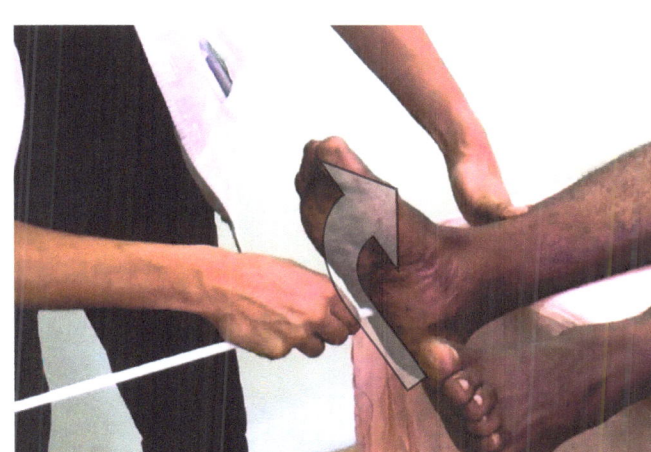

- What happens in normal people:
    - Flexion of big toe (called a flexor plantar response)
- What happens in UMN disease:
    - Triple Response
        - Toe comes up (points upwards, extends upwards)
        - Foot will come up (foot dorsiflexes)
        - Knee flexion (pulling the whole foot up)
    - Note: the up-going plantar reflex of the toe is usually the first sign of the triple response (i.e. you don't always see all three responses!)
    - Note: differentiate between patients who voluntarily retract their legs up because of the pain/ticklish sensation of the test compared to when you use a blunt object and it is a reflex!
    - Note: this is also known as the extensor plantar response OR Barbisnky Reflex and is always pathological!

Chapter 3

The Sensory System

- This system is divided according to the sensory tracks of the spine as follows:
    o Spinothalamic Tract
        - Temperature
        - Light touch
        - Pin prick
    o Posterior Column Tract
        - Joint Position Sense
        - Vibration

Introduction

- This examination is almost entirely subjective!
- Sensory loss can only occur on the skin
- On the skin sensory loss has to assume a certain shape
- **Therefore there are 2 questions one must answer during this examination:**
  - o **Is there sensory loss?**
  - o **What is the shape of the sensory loss?**

- Note: the shape will help you to localize the lesion!

- **General principles** of examining the sensory system (3 BASIC STEPS):

  - o Show patient what the sensation is like (normally) in an area that we know is normal from the history (this will establish the baseline)

  - o We then immediately go to the middle of the complained of area
    - ▪ Compare the sensation of this area with the exact same piece of skin on the other side of the body
    - ▪ If there is a difference then we have established that there is a sensory loss

  - o We then start from that area that is abnormal and we move out quickly to determine the shape of the sensory loss

Basic Physiology of the Sensory System

There are 2 types of sensation:

1.) Spinothalamic
- **Temperature**
- **Light touch**
- **Pin prick**

   Note 1: The Spinothalamic Tract **enters the spinal cord, immediately crosses the midline**, then ascends up to the brainstem, goes through the thalamus and then to the sensory cortex

   Note: 2: Temperature is hardly ever used during the examination and instead we look at light touch and pin prick to assess the spinothalamic tract

2.) Posterior Column Sensation
- **Joint position sensation**
- **Vibration**

   Note 1: The Posterior Column Tract enters the spinal cord, does not cross the midline, ascends up ipsilaterally, **enters the medulla and there is where it crosses over**, then it goes to the thalamus and then to the sensory cortex

- Note 2: all sensation ends up in the contralateral side of the brain (thalamus and cortex)

Light Touch:

2 techniques:
- **Cotton wool technique**
  - o This is the traditional method
  - o It is not the most accurate though

Procedure:

STEP 1
- o Take a small piece of cotton wool, and make small wisp at the end of it (i.e. don't just take the whole piece of cotton wool and use it like that!)

- o Explain to patient (with their eyes open) that you are going to touch them with the cotton wool and then touch them (on a normal area) to show them how it feels
  - ▪ Then ask patient to close their eyes!
  - ▪ Then go to an area that you know to be normal from the history and touch it with the cotton wool
  - ▪ Tell the patient that if they feel it they should say "yes"

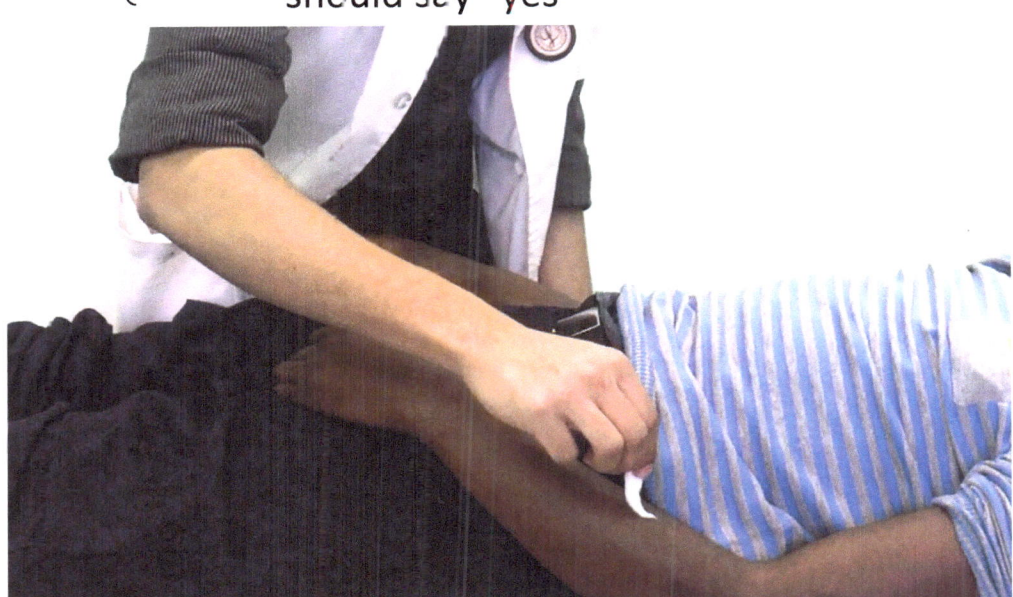

STEP 2

- o Now move on to the abnormal area
  - Start in the middle of the suspected abnormal area
  - With the patient's eyes still closed, see if the patient responds
- o Then move on to the same piece of the skin on the opposite side of the body
  - Lightly touch this skin and hear if this elicits a response
  - This will answer our 1st question – is there sensory loss

STEP 3

- o Determine the shape of the sensory loss
  - Simply jus fan out around the abnormal area, and touch the skin as many times as you like until the patient says "yes" thereby marking the borders of the sensory loss

- **Finger technique**
  - o Use your finger as the stimulus (instead of cotton wool)
  - o Advantage: stimulus is familiar, can discriminate character
    - Do you feel me touching you?
    - Does it feel like a finger?
  - o Therefore, if the patient says that they can feel your finger but it does not feel the same as the other side/ it does not feel like a finger, then it is an abnormal area and you need to use the 3 step approach (above) and determine the shape of the area affected!

Note: when checking light touch, one does not need to test every single dermatome! Simply just check anterior and posterior side of the:
- Hands
- Arms
- Trunk and back
- Legs

Pin Prick:

- 2 techniques:
  - **Traditional method – the sharp/blunt method**

    - Get a pin with a blunt end and a sharp end (DO NOT use a needle from the wards)

    STEP 1 {
    - Go to a known normal area of skin
      - Tell patient this is the sharp end and this is the blunt end (so that they are aware of how it feels)
    - Next, ask the patient to close their eyes
    - Then ask the patient which is the sharp end and which is the blunt end
      - Test the normal area again (this is to confirm that they can differentiate between the two)

    STEP 2 {
    - Now move onto the abnormal area
    - Check if they can differentiate between sharp and blunt
    - Compare left side from right
    - Basically establish if abnormal

    STEP 3 {
    - Fan out and determine shape

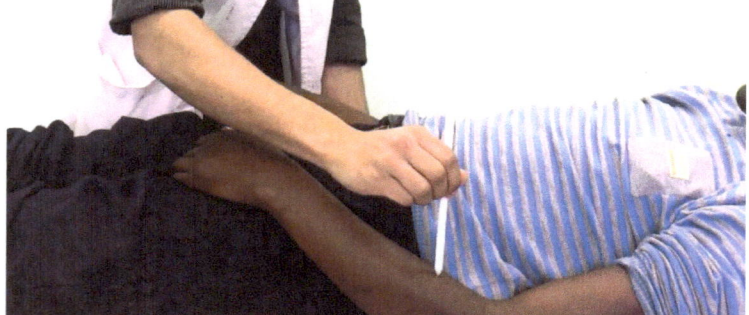

o **Toothpick method (basically a characteristic sharp method)**

- This is the same as the traditional method except for the following:
  - You do not use anything blunt
  - You must compare the behaviour of the patient of the one side's toothpick prick to the other.
  - In other words, the patient will say one side is more sharp than the other!

  - Note: ALWAYS go through the 3 step general principles when doing both methods!

Joint Position Sense:

- This is the only objective test in the sensory exam

- Procedure:
    - Aim: Move the toe up and down and elicit if the patient can determine which position the toe is in (whilst ensuring the patient closes their eyes)

    - Ensure that you hold the toe on the sides/laterally (DO NOT push the toe up from underneath, or down on the nail!)
    - Then explain to the patient what you are about to do:
        - "I am going to move your toe up and down, you must then close your eyes and tell me which way I am moving your toe in."
    - Initially be obvious about the movements and do large movements with the toe
        - This to ensure that the patient understands the game

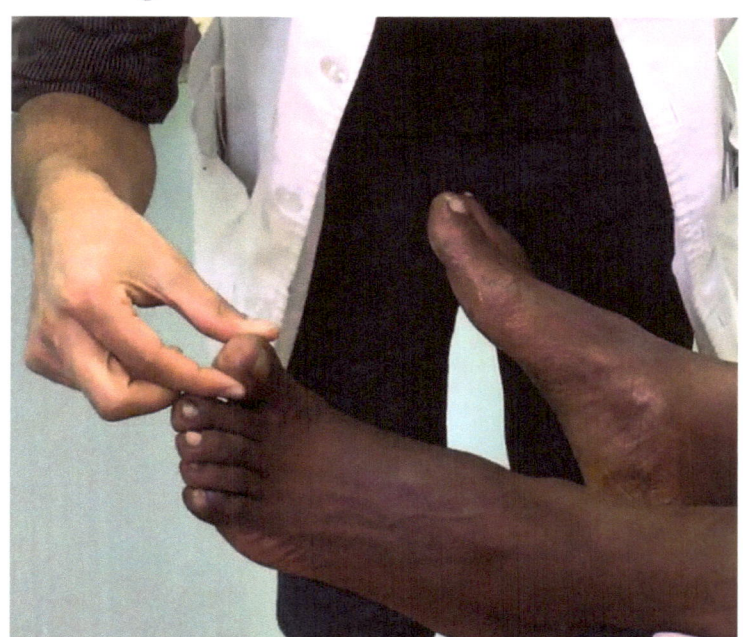

- o Next, you need to say that you are going to make the game a bit more difficult
  - This time you will be making far smaller movements with the toe
  - Normal: the slightest movement can be noticed
  - If the patient gets 3 answers in a row correct then they are normal

- Note: patients with joint position sense problems will most commonly have a problem with walking since joint position is required in order to walk.

Vibration:

- Use the tuning fork (usually 128Hz)
  - o Low frequency is what is required

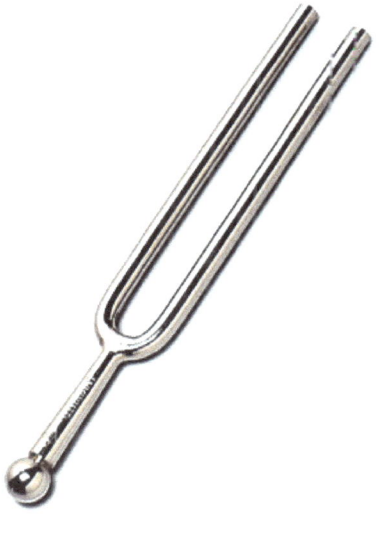

- Explain the game to the patient:
  - o Put tuning fork into motion (by flicking it gently)
    - Place by ear and tell patient if they hear it
    - Tell them we are NOT testing this sound
  - o Put tuning fork again into motion
    - Place onto the patient's clavicle
    - Ask them if they feel it
    - When they say yes, tell them that is what we're testing for!

- Procedure:
  o Put the tuning fork into motion
  o Place the vibrating fork onto a boney prominence
    ▪ E.g. medial malleolus
  o Ask patient if they feel it vibrating
  o If they do, ask them to say when it stops vibrating
    ▪ As soon as the patient says it stops vibrating, move it to the metacarpals (wrist)
    ▪ Then ask patient do they feel it now
      ● Normal: shouldn't feel it (i.e. vibration from metacarpals/wrist joint and from malleolus is about the same)
      ● Abnormal: if they feel it vibrating for a reasonable length of time in the metacarpals after having stopped feeling it in the medial malleolus
      ● Abnormal: if they don't feel it at all in the medial malleolus
        o The next step would be to move up the leg and determine at which point the vibration is felt best
        o If there is a gradient that is determined then it is most probably due to peripheral neuropathy
        o If there is a distinct area where it can be felt and a distinct area where it can't be felt then it may indicate spinal cord pathology at a certain level.

Chapter 4

The 12 Cranial Nerves (CN I-CN XII)

- Overview:
    - o There are 12 bilaterally paired cranial nerves
    - o These cranial nerves carry afferent and efferent fibres between the brain and peripheral structures (i.e. head and neck)
    - o The first two cranial nerves attach directly to the brain
    - o The rest of the cranial nerves have various nuclei within the brainstem

Mnemonic to remember the Cranial Nerves:

1	Oh	Olfactory	CN I
2	Oh	Optic	CN II
3	Oh	Occulomotor	CN III
4	To	Trochlear	CN IV
5	Touch	Trigeminal	CN V
6	And	Abducens	CN VI
7	Feel	Facial	CN VII
8	Various	Vestibulocochlear	CN VIII
9	Girls'	Glossopharyngeal	CN IX
10	Vaginas	Vagus	CN X
11	And	Accessory	CN XI
12	Hymen	Hypoglossal	CN XII

In this chapter we will only focus on the examination of each of these cranial nerves.

Cranial Nerve I – Olfactory nerve:

Anatomy:

- This is a purely sensory nerve

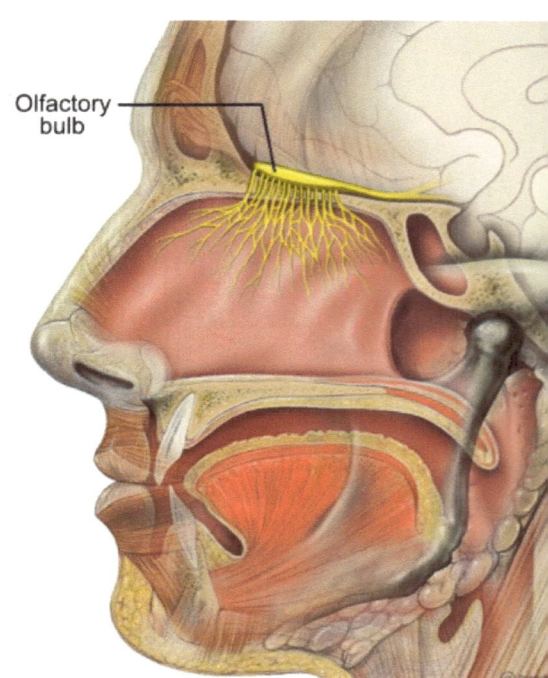

Olfactory bulb

- Fibres arise in the mucous membrane of the nose and pass through the cribriform plate of the ethmoid bone to synapse in the olfactory bulb.

Testing:

- <u>Not routinely tested</u>
  - o only if frontal lobe pathology suspected
- Test both perception and identification / recognition using aromatic non irritant material

- Close one nostril, whilst patient sniffs essences with other
- Use 2 different smells
- Ask patient to close eyes
- Let them smell both things
- Then test them by asking them to match which smell from the 2 that you gave are they smelling at a particular time (with their eyes closed of course)
- i.e. it will test their sense of smell and not their ability to name a smell!

Cranial Nerve II – Optic Nerve

Anatomy:

- It is a purely sensory nerve
- This nerve starts in the eye; it then passes through the optic foramen close to the ophthalmic artery and joins the optic nerve from the opposite side to form the optic chiasm. From this optic chiasm, it then splits again and goes to each half of the brain

- Fibres from the temporal visual fields (the nasal halves of the retinas) cross in the chiasm, whereas those from the nasal visual fields do not.

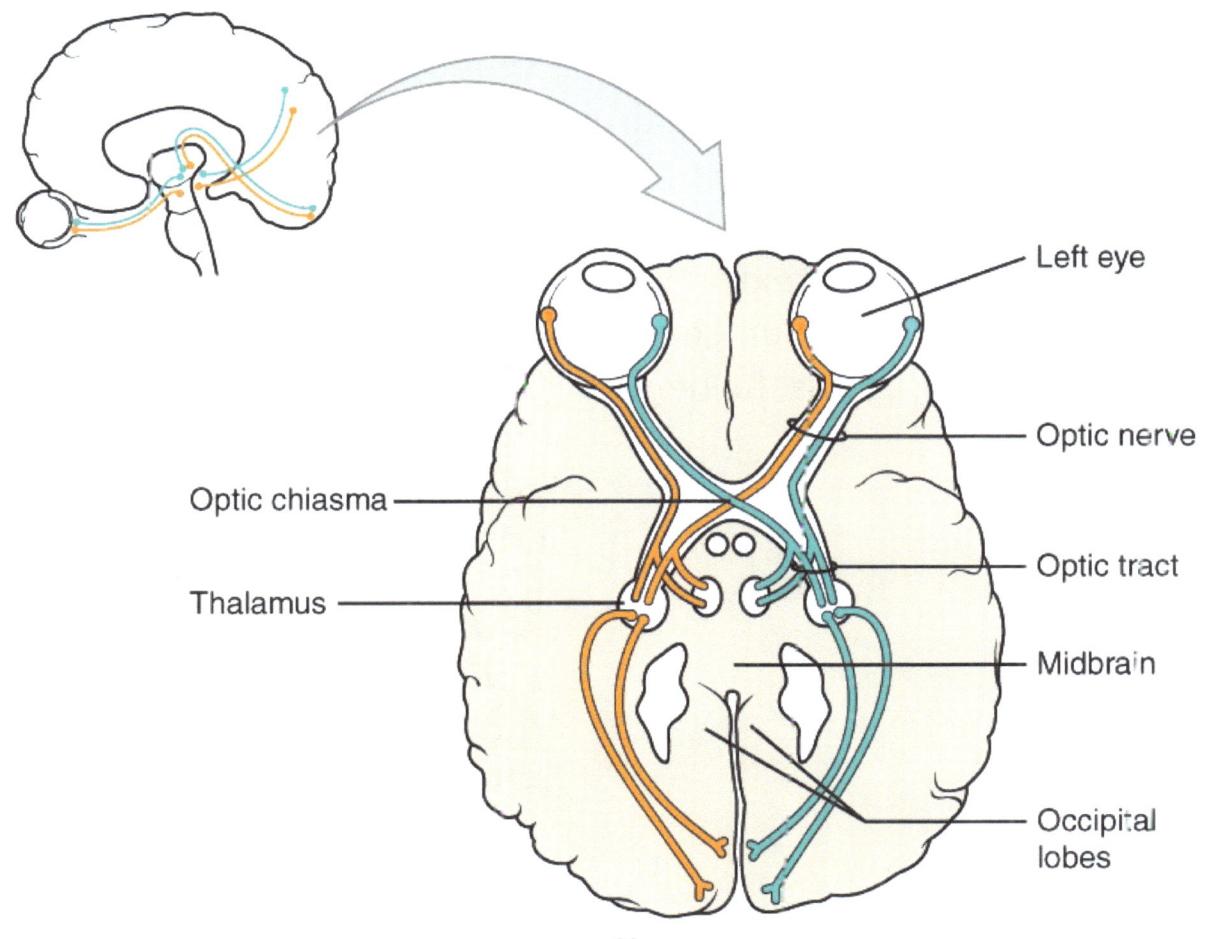

Left eye

Optic nerve

Optic chiasma

Optic tract

Thalamus

Midbrain

Occipital lobes

Testing the Optic Nerve (CN II):

- There are 4 components to test for:
  1.) Visual Acuity
    - Tests central vision
  2.) Visual Fields
    - Tests peripheral vision
  3.) Pupils
  4.) Fundoscopy

1.) Visual Acuity:
  a. Light
      i. Can they see if light from torch is on or off?
  b. Hand movements
      i. Do they see your hand moving (side to side or up and down?)
  c. **Finger Counting** (usually tests light and hand movements automatically)
      i. **How many fingers am I holding up?**
  d. **Reading text**
      i. Snellen Chart is useful here

	E	1	20/200
F	P	2	20/100
T O Z		3	20/70
L P E D		4	20/50
P E C F D		5	20/40
E D F C Z P		6	20/30
F E L O P Z D		7	20/25
D E F P O T E C		8	20/20
L E F O D P C T		9	
F D P L T C E O		10	
P E Z O L C F T D		11	

2.) Visual Fields:

- o Patient covers one eye with their hand
- o Patient looks straight ahead
- o Examiner keeps his hand ½ way between the patient and himself
- o Examiner closes same side of his eye as the patient
- o Check the following quadrants:
    1. upper quadrant
    2. equator
    3. lower quadrant
- o Check by moving/wiggling finger and asking patient to point to which hand is moving (in all 3 quadrants on both sides)

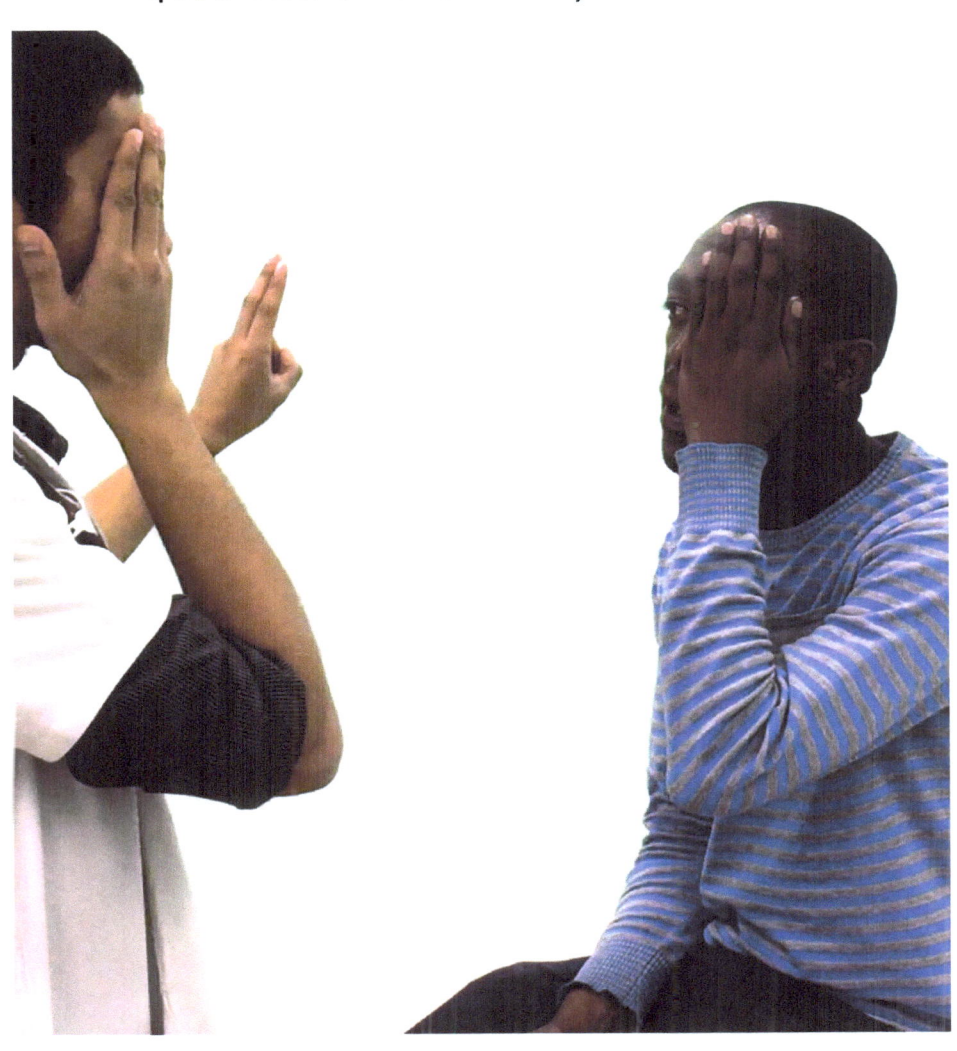

3.) Pupils:

- Constriction to light (afferent fibres)
  - o Direct
    - ■ This can be checked by bringing a light from the side of a patient's head and shining it at the pupil
    - ■ The direct response is normal if the pupil constricts
  - o Consensual (this is actually a function of CN III, but can be checked at this point already)
    - ■ This is checked by looking at the opposite eye when shining the light
    - ■ If both eyes constrict when light is shone into one eye then the consensual response is present and normal

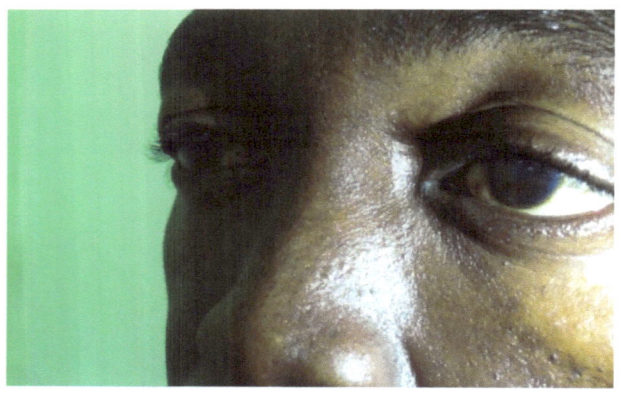

Top Tip: DO NOT shine light directly into eye from the front (otherwise the patient will accommodate to the near object and you will not be testing the light reflex)! INSTEAD shine the light into the eye from the side!

4.) Fundoscopy:

- Use a fundoscope to assess the eye
- This is not routinely done during the neurological examination
- It is particularly useful when suspecting raised intra cranial pressure
  - o This will be seen as papilloedema during fundoscopy

Cranial Nerve III – Occulomotor Nerve

Anatomy:

Note: Cranial Nerves III, IV, and VI are all involved in the control of eye movement
We will therefore look at them together

- The oculomotor nerve (CN III) carries the majority of somatic motor neurones that innervate extraocular muscles and is therefore responsible for moving the eye (in almost all its directions)

- The oculomotor Nerve supplies and innervates:
  - **All the extraocular muscles EXCEPT**
    - **Superior oblique (CN IV)**
    - **Lateral rectus (CN VI)**
  - Therefore the oculomotor nerve causes the eye to:
    - Elevate
    - Depress
    - Adduct (or move medially)
    - But it can't cause the eye to move
      - Down and in (Superior Oblique/CN IV)
      - Laterally (Lateral Rectus/CN IV)

- Important Note:
  - CN III also has the function for the papillary light reflex (as described for CN II), but the difference is that CN II is responsible for afferent fibres and CN III for efferent fibres of this reflex

Testing:

- <mark>Simply ask patient to face forward and then with their eyes follow your fingers as you make an "H" shape so that you check all movements of the eye</mark>

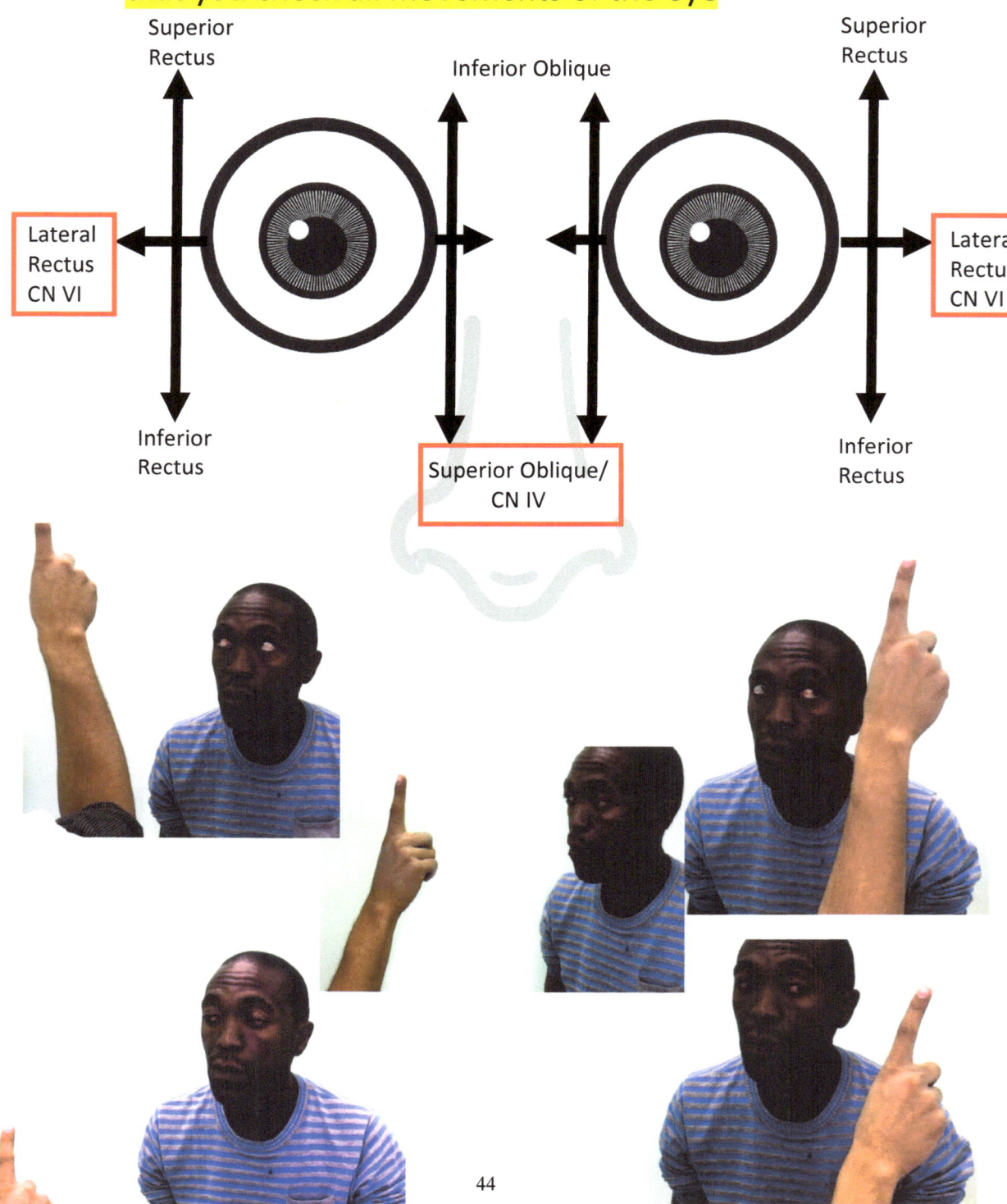

Superior Rectus

Inferior Oblique

Superior Rectus

Lateral Rectus CN VI

Lateral Rectus CN VI

Inferior Rectus

Superior Oblique/ CN IV

Inferior Rectus

CN IV: Trochlear Nerve:

- This nerve contain only somatic motor neurones
- Its only function is to innervate the **superior oblique muscle** (of the eye)

- This then supplies the superior oblique muscle
- This muscle allows the eyeball to move downwards and medially

CN VI: Abducens Nerve:

- This nerve contain only somatic motor neurones (just like the trochlear)
- Its only function is to innervate the **lateral rectus** (of the eye)

- This then supplies the lateral rectus muscle
- This muscle allows the eyeball to abduct (∴ the name of the nerve is ABDUCens)

CN V: Trigeminal Nerve

Anatomy:

- The trigeminal nerve has 2 components:
    o A sensory component
    o A motor component
- It is the main sensory nerve for the head
- It also innervates the muscles of mastication as well

- **Sensory component:**
    o The trigeminal nerve has 3 peripheral branches:
        ▪ An ophthalmic nerve
        ▪ A maxillary nerve
        ▪ A mandibular nerve

- **Motor component:**
    o Supplies/Innervates:
        ▪ Muscles of mastication
            • Masseter
            • Temporalis   } Closes the jaw
            • Lateral and
              medial pteryogoids } Opens the jaw

Testing CN V:

- There are 4 things to check:
    - o Corneal Reflex
    - o Sensation
    - o Motor Division
    - o Jaw Jerk

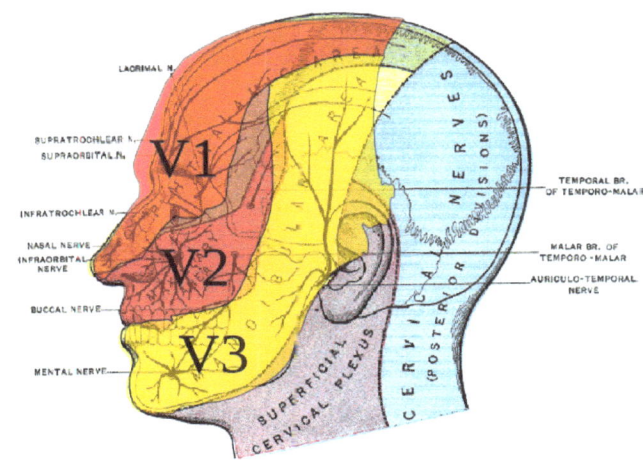

- Corneal Reflex:
    - o Lightly touch the cornea (*not* the conjunctiva) with a wisp of cotton wool brought to the eye from the side.
    - o Reflex blinking of *both* eyes is a normal response.

- Sensation:
    - o Test *facial sensation* in the three divisions of the nerve, comparing each side with the other:
        - Opthalmic Area (V1)
        - Maxillary Area (V2)
        - Mandibular Area (V3)
    - o Test first with the sharp end of a new neurological pin for pain sensation.
    - o The patient keeps the eyes closed and a new piece of cottonwool is used to test light touch in the same way
    - o Ensure that you can identify the regions on the face! I.e. sensation from trigeminal stops infront of ear and does not go to angle of jaw!

- **Motor Division:**
  o The motor division involves muscles of chewing
  o Inspect for wasting of the temporal and masseter muscles

  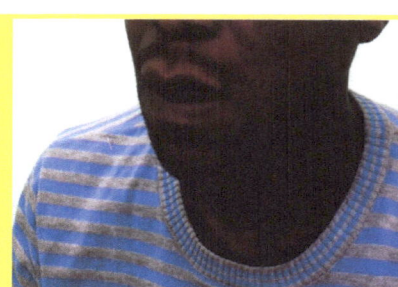

  1. **Masseter muscle**
     "Please clench your teeth"
     (then feel infront of ear)

  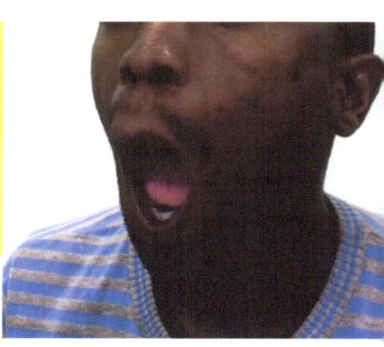

  2. **Pterygoid**
     "Please move your jaw side to side"
     (will deviate to abnormal side)

  3. **Temporalis**
     " Please open your jaw/mouth"
     (then try and close the jaw)

- **Jaw Jerk:**
  o Test the *jaw jerk* or *masseter reflex*
  o The patient lets the mouth fall open slightly and the examiner's finger is placed on the tip of the jaw/chin area
  o This is then tapped lightly with a tendon hammer
  o Normally there is a slight closure of the mouth or no reaction at all.
  o In an upper motor neurone (UMN) lesion above the pons the jaw jerk is greatly exaggerated.
  o This is commonly seen in pseudobulbar palsy

CN VII: Facial Nerve

Anatomy:
- The facial nerve contains 3 components:
    o Sensory component
    o Motor component
    o Parasympathetic component

Sensory Fibres:
- Receives input from:
    o **Taste sensation from:**
        ▪ Anterior 2/3rds of tongue
        ▪ Floor of the mouth
        ▪ Soft palate
    o **Cutaneous sensation from:**
        ▪ Part of the external ear

Motor fibres:
- Supplies/Innervates:
    o The **muscles of facial expression**
    o A muscle of the **middle ear**

Pathology:
- **An upper motor neurone (UMN) lesion** will cause lower facial nerve paralysis only!
- This is because the forehead would be supplied bilaterally so will not be paralysed as it is still innervated
- **A lower motor neurone (LMN) lesion** will cause complete paralysis of the affected side as it would have essentially cut off any supply to the affected side

Testing CN VII:

- In order to test the muscles of facial expression, ask the patient to do the following:

1.) "Look Up"
- Check for wrinkling of the forehead
- If this is absent it may indicate an UMN facial nerve palsy

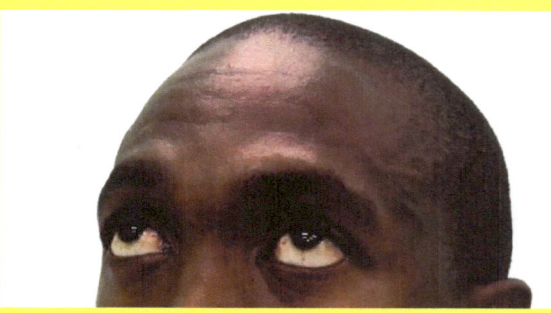

2.) "Close your eyes tightly" (check for buried eyelashes)

(DO NOT try and open it with your thumb!)

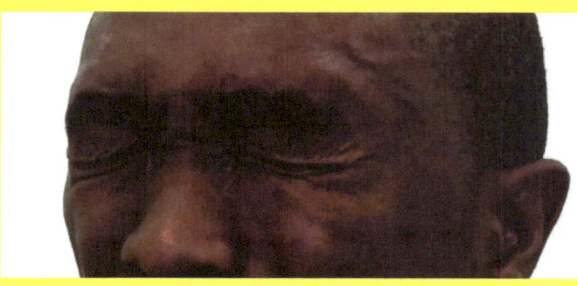

3.) "Blow up your cheeks like a balloon"

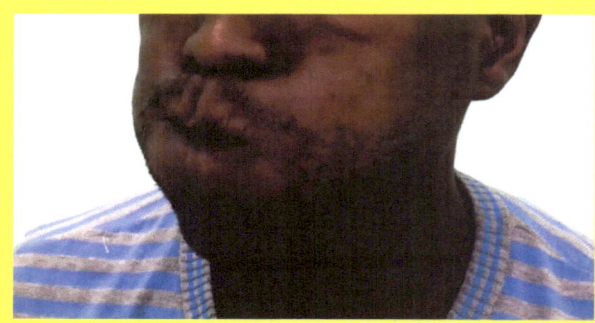

4.) "Show me your teeth"

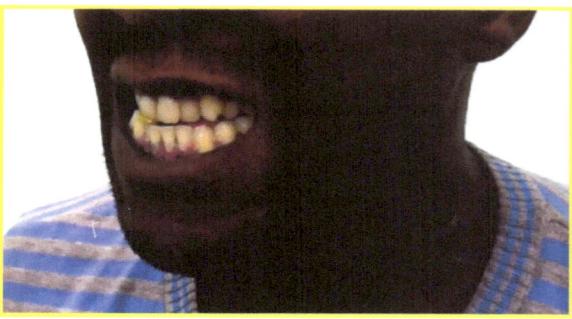

A Note of Facial Nerve Palsy:

- It is important to note that the facial nerve has bilateral supply (from the brain) for the forehead and unilateral supply (from the brain) to the rest of the face
- The pattern of how a facial nerve palsy looks is determined by one question:
  - Is it an UMN lesion or a LMN lesion?

Upper Motor Neuron Lesion	Lower Motor Neuron Lesion
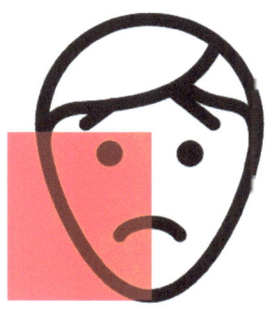	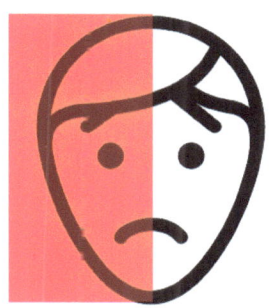
- The key point to note is that there is forehead sparing i.e. the forehead of someone with an UMN lesion of CN VII has wrinkling of their forehead - The rest of the affected side of the face, though, is weak and droops down	- The key point to note is that the forehead IS affected as well i.e. the forehead of someone with an LMN lesion of CN VII has no wrinkling of their forehead on the affected side! - Therefore the entire affected side of the face is weak and droops down

CN VIII: Vestibulocochlear Nerve

Anatomy:

- This is a sensory nerve (only!)
- This nerve has 2 components:
  - o **Vestibular nerve**
    - ▪ This carries information related to position and movement of the head
    - ▪ Receives input from:
      - • Hair cells of the vestibular portion of the membranous labyrinth
  - o **Cochlear nerve**
    - ▪ This carries auditory information
    - ▪ Receives input from:
      - • Hair cells of the Organ of Corti (in the inner ear)

Top Tip:
Crude way to check hearing:

Simply ask patient if they can hear this:
Rub some hair strands between your fingers next to their ear.
Note: elderly people have physiological hearing loss and may not be able to hear this.

Testing CN VIII:

- Rinne's Test
  - ○ In **Rinné's test** a 256 Hz vibrating tuning fork is placed on the mastoid process, behind the ear, and when the sound is no longer heard it is placed in line with the external meatus
  - ○ Normally the note is audible at the external meatus.
  - ○ **In nerve deafness both air and bone conduction are diminished.**
  - ○ **In conduction deafness bone conduction is better than air conduction.**

- Weber's Test
  - ○ In **Weber's test** a vibrating 256 Hz tuning fork is positioned on the centre of the forehead.
  - ○ Normally the sound is heard in the centre of the forehead.
  - ○ **Nerve deafness causes the sound to be heard better in the normal ear.**
  - ○ Conduction deafness causes the sound to be louder in the abnormal ear

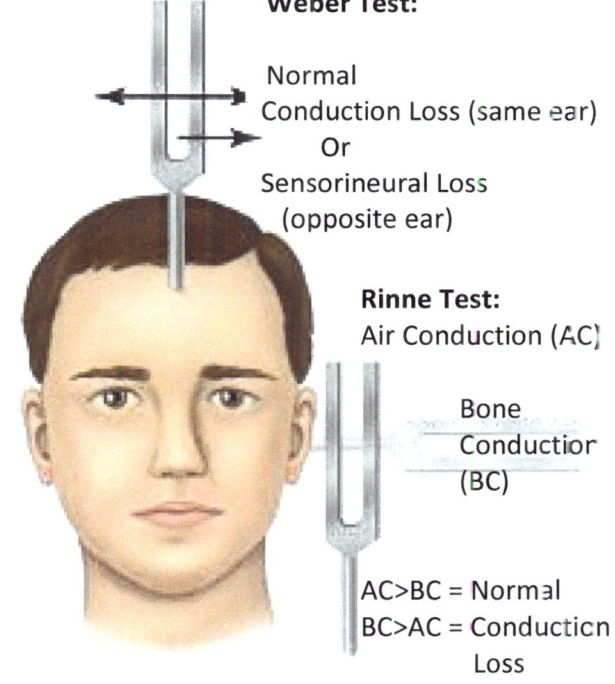

Weber Test:

Normal
Conduction Loss (same ear)
Or
Sensorineural Loss
(opposite ear)

Rinne Test:
Air Conduction (AC)

Bone
Conduction
(BC)

AC>BC = Normal
BC>AC = Conduction Loss

CN IX: Glossopharyngeal Nerve

- This is mainly a sensory nerve
- BUT it also has a few motor fibres and parasympathetic fibres

Sensory Component:
- Receives input from:
  o General sensation of the pharynx (tastebuds), posterior 1/3 of the tongue, eustachian tube, and middle ear
  o Chemoreceptors in the carotid body and baroreceptors in the carotid sinus

Motor component:
- Supplies/innervates:
  o Stylopharyngeus muscle (this is involved in swallowing)

Note:
Testing of CN IX and CN X is ALWAYS done together

CN X: Vagus Nerve

- This nerve has 3 components:
  - o Sensory component
  - o Motor component
  - o Parasympathetic component

Sensory component:
- Receives input from:
  - o General sensation of:
    - Pharynx
    - Larynx
    - Oesophagus
    - Tympanic membrane
    - External auditory meatus
    - Part of the concha of the external ear
  - o Chemoreceptors in the aortic bodies and baroreceptors in the aortic arch
  - o Receptors widely distributed throughout the thoracic and abdominal viscera

Motor component:
- Supplies/Innervates:
  - o Soft palate
  - o Pharynx
  - o Larynx
  - o Upper part of the oesophagus

Testing of CN IX and X:

Note: we ALWAYS clinically examine CN IX and X together!

- Palate
    - Check for nasal speech
- Pharynx:
    - Check for dysphagia
        - Difficulty swallowing may be due to CN IX and X pathology
        - Simply ask patient to swallow
- Larynx
    - Voice disturbances
    - Weak cough (therefore ask patient to cough and if they can't do it forcefully it may indicate weakness)
- Displacement of the uvula
    - Ask patient to say "aaaaah" and inspect the palate with a torch
    - Note any displacement of the uvula
    - If the uvula is drawn to one side this indicates a unilateral tenth nerve palsy
        - *The uvula is drawn towards the NORMAL side in this case*
        - This is also known as the curtain sign (because the weak side droops down like a curtain)
- Gag Reflex:
    - Reflex contraction of back of throat and is evoked by touching the roof of the mouth
    - Afferent sensation of gag reflex is supplied by CN IX and efferent is supplied by CN X

CN XI: Accessory Nerve:

Anatomy:
- This nerve is a motor nerve (only!)
- It consists of two parts:
  - Cranial part
  - Spinal part

- Cranial Part supplies/innervates:
  - Soft palate
  - Pharynx
  - Larynx

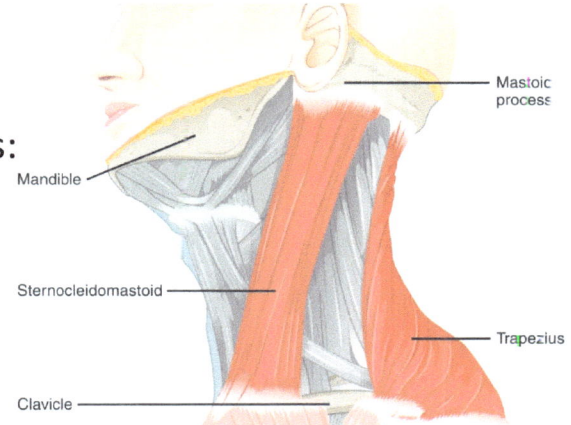

- Spinal Part supplies/innervates:
  - Sternocleidomastoid muscle
  - Trapezius muscle
- Note: These muscles function to move the head and shoulders

Testing the Accessory Nerve:

Trapezius Muscle: "Lift up your shoulders"

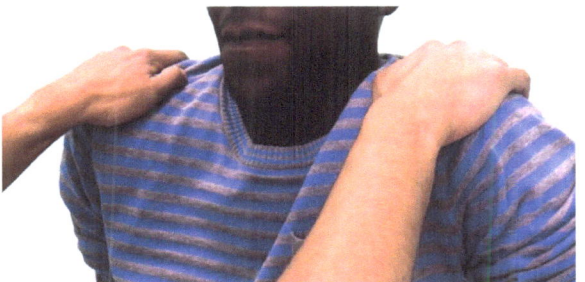

Sternocleidomastoid muscle: "turn your head to the side"

(Look at the muscle and check for wasting as well)

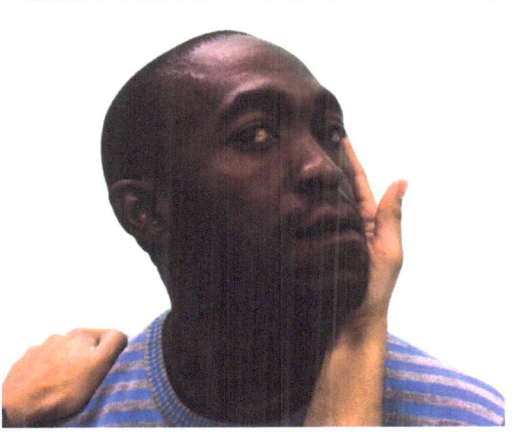

CN XII: Hypoglossal Nerve

Anatomy:
- This is a motor nerve (only!)

- It supplies two main components of the tongue:
  o Extrinsic components
  o Intrinsic components
- Therefore it serves to both:
  o move the tongue
  o change the shape of the tongue

Testing the Hypoglossal Nerve:
- Ask the patient to poke out the tongue

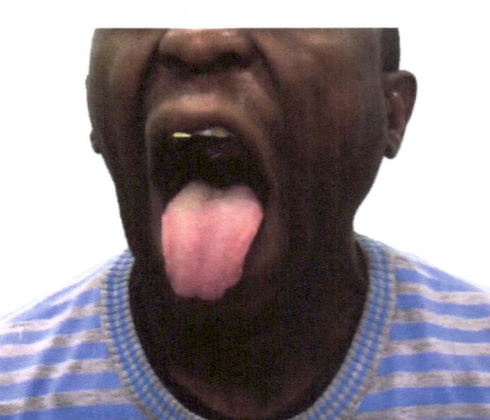

- It may *deviate towards the weaker (affected) side if there is a unilateral **lower motor neuron** lesion.*
- The tongue, like the face and palate, has a bilateral upper motor neuron innervation in most people, so a unilateral upper motor neuron lesion often causes no deviation.

- Also check tongue for:
  o Fasciculations
  o Wasting
  o Power (ask the patient to push their tongue against their cheek and you apply some resistance to assess the power)

Chapter 5

The Cerebellar System

<u>Overview of the Cerebellar System</u>

Function of the Cerebellar System:
- Provides the body with coordination
- Note: proximal muscles is what give you cerebellar control
    - o As opposed to peripheral fine motor movement which is highly skilled corticospinal movements

Approach to pathology:
There are 2 main syndromes:
- Central (vermal) Cerebellar Syndrome
    - o Hallmark: truncal ataxia
        - ▪ Balancing your top half with your bottom half
- Lateral (hemispheral) Cerebellar Syndrome
    - o Hallmark: ipsilateral limb ataxia

- Associated signs for both:
    - o Nystagmus
    - o Cerebellar dysarthria

Mnemonic to remember the cerebellar signs is:

	Sign:	Testing:
D	Dysdiadochokinesis	Tapping one hand onto the other, whilst alternating between tapping the palm and the dorsum
A	Ataxia	Heel-to-shin test Finger nose test (past pointing)
S	Slurred speech	"PTK" test
H	Hypotonia	Check for tone
I	Intention tremor	Finger Nose Test
N	Nystagmus	Check the eyes
G	Gait abnormality	Walk normally and then walk with one foot infront of other

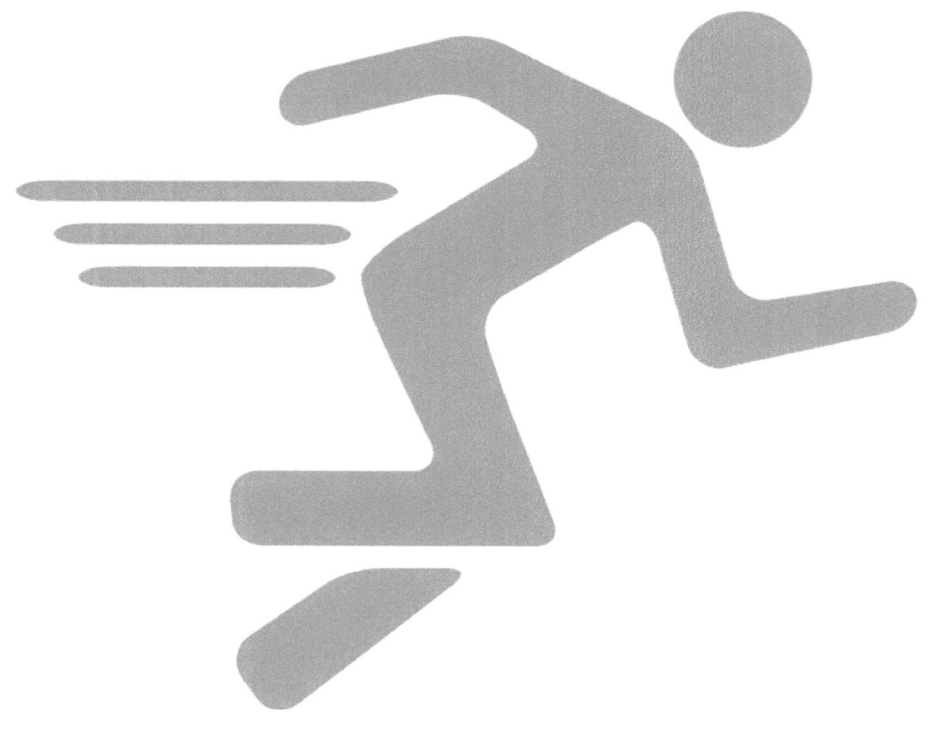

==Testing Limb Ataxia:==

==Upper Limb:==
- Finger- Nose Test
  o Ask the patient to place their finger on their nose
  o ENSURE that the patient's arm is held up parallel to the ground
  o Then ask the patient to touch your finger
  o Check both arms with the finger-nose test

  o Look for the following abnormlaities:
    ▪ ==intention tremor==, which is a tremor that increases as the target is approached (there is no tremor at rest)
    ▪ past-pointing==/dysmetria (inability to estimate distance)==
      • The patient's finger overshoots the target towards the side of cerebellar abnormality

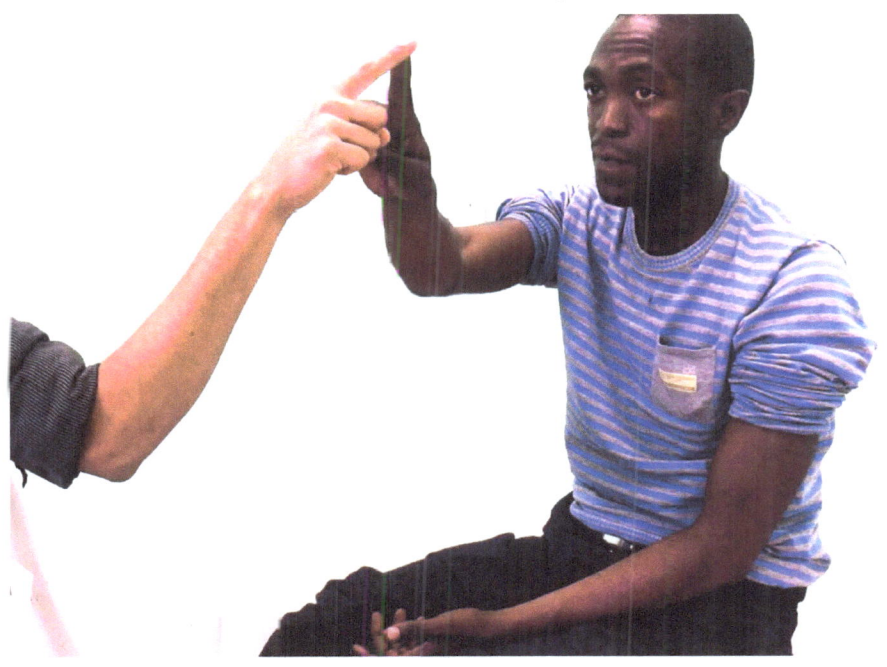

- ==Tapping Hands==
  - Ask patient to hit the palm of 1 hand with the palm of the other hand
    - This should be regular and rhythmical
    - If it is not then there is limb ataxia
  - Once again, the patients arm should be parallel to the ground

- ==Tap and turn hands==
  - This is similar to the above test except instead of just tapping the hands the patient has to alternatively turn the tapping hand
  - The inability to do so is known as ==DYSDIADOCHOKINESIS== (DDK)

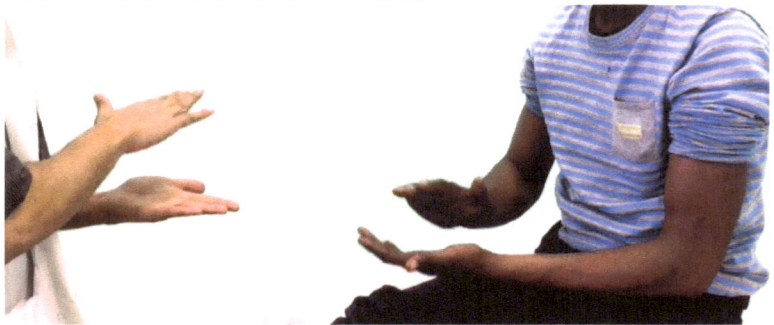

==Lower Limb:==
- ==Heel-Shin Test:==
  - Ask patient to put their one heel on the opposite side's knee
  - Then ask to run the heel down the tibia/leg
  - Test both legs

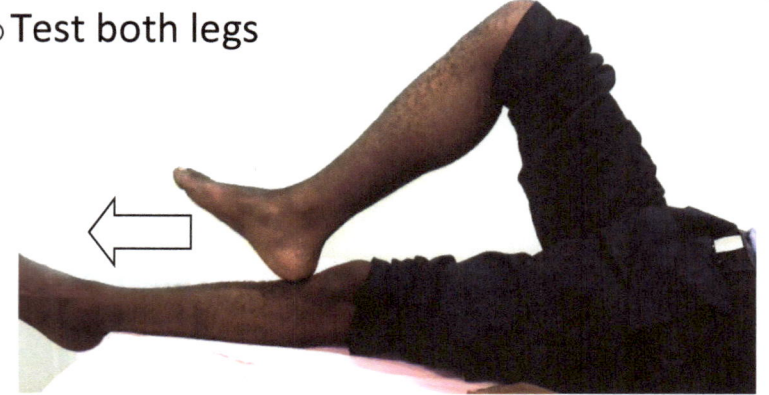

Walking/ Heel-to-toe walking

- This tests for an ataxic gait
- Ask patient to walk normally
- Then ask patient to walk with 1 foot in front of the other in a heel-to-toe manner (also known as tandem walking)

- In both cases if there is cerebellar dysfunction:
    - o Patient can't do the activity at all
    - o Note: the patient is allowed to wobble and use the hands to balance, but they must be able to do the activity!

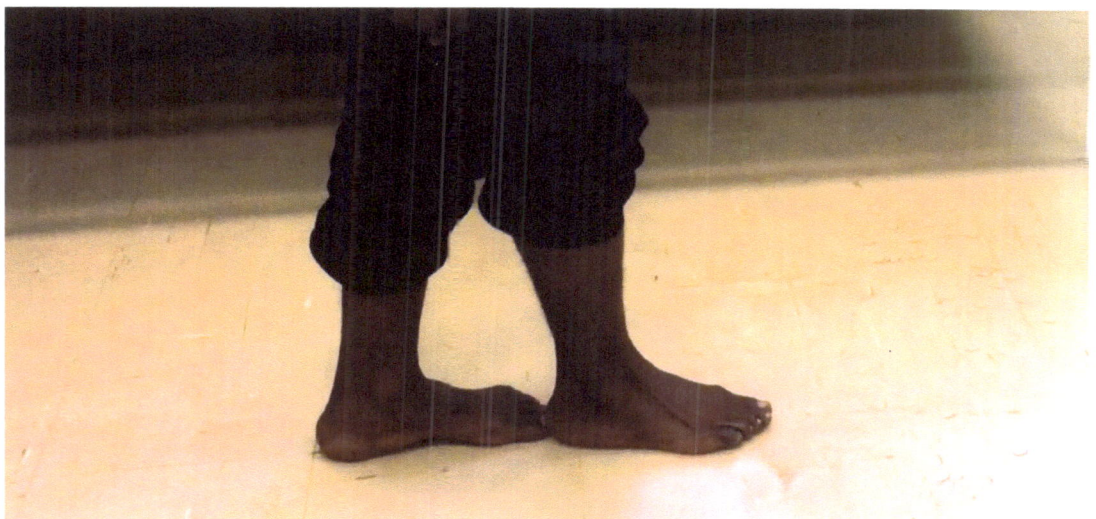

About turn

- Whilst the patient is walking, ask them to turn 180 degrees and face the opposite the direction
- Check this when the patient turns right and when the patient turns left

Associated signs:

- Nystagmus:
  o Involuntary jerky horizontal movement of both eyes with an increased amplitude on looking towards the side of the lesion
  o This is prominent when asking the patient to look left and assessing for the movement and then asking to look right and assessing for the movement

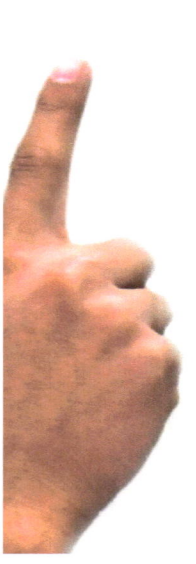 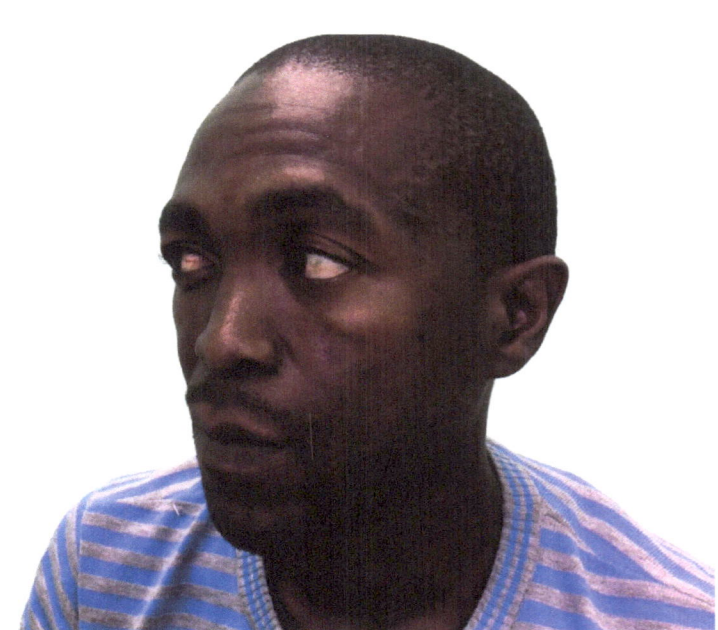

- Cerebellar Dysarthria:
  o Ask the patient to repeat:
    ▪ "P P P" "T T T" "K K K"
  o Then
    ▪ "PeTeKe PeTeKe"
  o Check for slurred speech

Summary:

Mental State Exam:
- GCS (?/15) ($E_3V_4M_5$)
- MMSE (if required)

Motor Exam:
- **Tone:**
  - UL:
    - Supination and pronation of arm
    - Wrist circumduction
    - Flexion and extension of UL
  - LL:
    - Log Rolling the leg
    - Lifting the leg quickly up under the knee
    - Checking for clonus
- **Power:**
  - UL:
    - Shrug shoulders
    - Flex arms
    - Extend arms
    - 2 finger grip
    - Fingers abducted
  - LL:
    - Hip flexion
    - Knee extension
    - Dorsiflexion of ankle (point foot upwards)
    - Big toe extension
    - Plantar flexion (point foot downwards)
  - Abdominal:
    - Ask patient to bring head off the bed (thus tensing rectus abdominus muscles)
- **Reflexes:**
  - UL:
    - Biceps reflex
    - Triceps reflex
    - Brachioradialis reflex
  - LL:
    - Knee reflex
    - Ankle Reflex
    - Babinsky/Plantar

Sensory Exam:

- **Cotton wool technique**
    - o Make a wisp of cotton a touch the patient
- **Finger technique**
    - o Check:
        - ▪ Hands, arms, trunk and back, legs
        - ▪ Anterior and posterior

- **Joint Position Sense**
    - o Check toes

- **Vibration**
    - o Tuning fork onto medial malleolus

Cerebellar Exam:

- DDK
    - o Tapping hands
    - o Tapping and turning
- Heel to shin test
- Finger nose test
- Heel to toe walking
- Check for nystagmus

Cranial Nerve Exam:

CN 2
- VA: Finger counting
- Visual Fields: 3 quadrants on each side
- Pupils: Direct and consensual light reflex

CN 3,4,6
- Follow fingers in H motion

CN 5
- Corneal reflex to cotton wool
- Sensation in 3 branches
- Clench teeth, move jaw side to side, open mouth
- Jaw jerk

CN 7:
- Look up for forehead wrinkling
- Blow up cheeks into balloon
- Show teeth

CN 8:
- Crude Test or Rinne/Weber tests

CN9, 10:
- Say aaah and check uvula

CN 11:
- Lift up shoulders
- Turn head side to side

CN 12:
- Ask patient to poke out tongue

If you enjoyed this book, and want similar titles in the future, simply leave us a review online, sign up to our Facebook page and let us know what topics you would like clarity on. We will get our minions to work on unconfusing any topic for you. After all, this is...

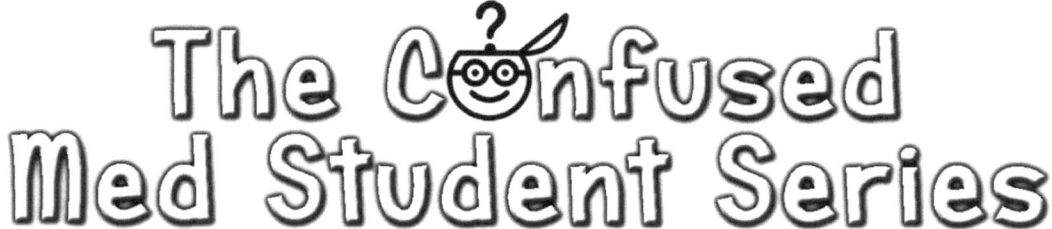

First Published, 2016

Although the author has made every effort to
ensure that the information in this book is
correct, the author does not assume and hereby
disclaim any liability to any party for any loss,
damage, or disruption caused by errors or
omissions, whether such errors or omissions
result from negligence, accident, or any other
cause.

www.ingramcontent.com/pod-product-compliance
Lightning Source LLC
Chambersburg PA
CBHW050855180526
45159CB00007B/2682